HIV/AIDS
NURSING
SECRETS

HIV/AIDS NURSING SECRETS

Judy K. Shaw, MS, ACRN, ANP-C
Section of Infectious Disease
Samuel S. Stratton VA Hospital
Albany, New York

Elizabeth Anne Mahoney, RN, MSN, EdD, ACRN
Professor of Nursing
Department of Nursing
The Sage Colleges
Troy, New York

Nursing Secrets Series Editor

Linda J. Scheetz, EdD, RN, CS, CEN
Assistant Professor, College of Nursing
Rutgers, The State University of New Jersey
Newark, New Jersey

HANLEY & BELFUS, INC./Philadelphia

Publisher: HANLEY & BELFUS, INC.
              Medical Publishers
              210 South 13th Street
              Philadelphia, PA 19107
              (215) 546-7293; 800-962-1892
              FAX (215) 790-9330
              Web site: http://www.hanleyandbelfus.com

Note to the reader: Although the techniques, ideas, and information in this book have been carefully reviewed for correctness, the authors, editors, and publisher cannot accept any legal responsibility for any errors or omissions that may be made. Neither the publisher nor the editors make any guarantee, expressed or implied, with respect to the material contained herein.

This book is designed to provide information about the background and modalities used frequently in HIV/AIDS nursing and how they are applied by practitioners in the field. It is not intended to be exhaustive, nor should patients use it as a substitute for the advice of their physician. It is strongly recommended that you talk with your own physician about any treatments you use personally, and research the area further for safety as it applies to the person you are treating. Before trying/recommending any treatment, the reader should review dosages, accepted indications, and other information pertinent to the safe and effective use of the therapies described.

Library of Congress Control Number: 2002112413

HIV/AIDS NURSING SECRETS   ISBN 1-56053-527-X

Last digit is the print number: 9   8   7   6   5   4   3   2   1

CONTENTS

CONTRIBUTORS

Brian D. Arey, MSN, ANP-BC
Nicholas A. Rango HIV Clinical Scholar, Division of HIV Medicine, Albany Medical Center, Albany, New York

Sandra A. Averitt, PhD, RN, LCCE
Associate Professor, Department of Nursing, Kennesaw State University, Kennesaw, Georgia

Mary Anne Brown, RN, BSN, MA
Program Director, Ryan White Title III Early Intervention Services, Hudson Headwaters Health Network, Glenn Falls, New York

Madeline Bronaugh, RN, MSN, ACRN
Affiliated Professor, Department of Nursing, Xavier University, Cincinnati, Ohio; Nurse Clinician, Infectious Disease Center, University Health Alliance, Cincinnati, Ohio

Inge B. Corless, RN, PhD, FAAN
Professor, Graduate Program in Nursing, Massachusetts General Hospital Institute of Health Professions, Boston, Massachusetts

Rosanna F. DeMarco, PhD, RN, ACRN
Assistant Professor, William F. Connell School of Nursing, Boston College, Chestnut Hill, Massachusetts

Pamela J. Dole, EdD, MPH, FNP, ACRN
Assistant Professor, Hunter-Bellevue School of Nursing, Hunter College, New York, New York

Richard S. Ferri, PhD, ANP, ACRN, FAAN
HIV/AIDS Nurse Practitioner, Provincetown, Massachusetts

Dale S. Ford, RN, MPH, CIC
Department of Infection Control, Yale University, New Haven, Connecticut; Massachusetts General Hospital, Boston, Massachusetts

Deborah M. Frank, ACRN, MS, ANP-C
AIDS Center, Department of Infectious Disease, University of Rochester, Rochester, New York

Donna M. Gallagher, RNCS, MS, ANP, FAAN
Assistant Professor, Office of Community Programs, University of Massachusetts Medical School and Graduate School of Nursing, Boston, Massachusetts; Nurse Practitioner, Mt. Auburn Hospital, Cambridge, Massachusetts

Minda J. Hubbard, MSN, RNC, ANP-C
Clinical Research Coordinator, HIV Medicine, Albany Medical Center, Albany, New York

Christine Johnsen, MPH, RN, CS
Health Promotion and Education Specialist, Center for Wellness and Health Communication, Harvard University Health Services, Cambridge, Massachusetts

Jeanne K. Kemppainen, PhD, RN
Associate Professor, School of Nursing, University of North Carolina at Wilmington, Wilmington, North Carolina

Elizabeth Anne Mahoney, RN, MSN, EdD, ACRN
Professor of Nursing, Department of Nursing, The Sage Colleges, Troy, New York

Patrice K. Nicholas, RN, DNSc, ANP, MPH
Associate Professor, Graduate Program in Nursing, Massachusetts General Hospital Institute of Health Professions, Boston, Massachusetts

Diane Nielsen, RN, BScN
Program Coordinator, Safeworks Calgary, Calgary Health Region, Calgary, Alberta, Canada

San Patten, MSc
Department of Community Health Services, University of Alberta, Calgary, Alberta, Canada

Judy K. Shaw, MS, ACRN, ANP-C
Section of Infectious Disease, Samuel S. Stratton VA Hospital, Albany, New York

Richard L. Sowell, PhD, RN, FAAN
Professor and Dean, College of Health and Human Services, Kennesaw State University, Kennesaw, Georgia

Lyn Stevens, MS, ACRN, NP
HIV Training Coordinator, HIV Clinical Education Initiative, New York State Department of Health AIDS Institute, State University of New York Upstate Medical University, Designated AIDS Center, Syracuse, New York

Adele A. Webb, PhD, RN, ACRN, FAAN
Executive Director, Association of Nurses in AIDS Care, Akron, Ohio

Yolanda Y. Wess, RN, BSN
Senior Research Assistant, Internal Medicine and Infectious Diseases, University of Cincinnati, Cincinnati, Ohio; Continuous Quality Improvement Coordinator, Infectious Disease Center, University Health Alliance, Cincinnati, Ohio

Vi Wilkes, MA, MS, ACRN
Faculty Facilitator and Trainer, University of Phoenix OnLine, Phoenix, Arizona

Kenneth Zwolski, RN, EdD, FNP-CS
Professor, School of Nursing, College of New Rochelle, New Rochelle, New York

PREFACE

HIV/AIDS is a pandemic that continues to proliferate despite therapeutic interventions that have changed the course of the disease from an acute to a chronic illness over the past 20 years. HIV/AIDS is nondiscriminatory and affects people of all ages, races, religions, and sexual orientations—directly, as people with the disease and their family, significant others, friends, and health care providers, or indirectly, as taxpayers forced to shoulder the burden of increasing health care costs and elected officials facing the possible loss of their workforce as the morbidity and mortality rates continue their upward spiral.

Working with actual or potential clients with HIV/AIDS (including families and significant others) provides nurses with unique and challenging experiences and opportunities. We must always remember that all clients are at risk for acquiring HIV/AIDS. Our role is to help them minimize that risk or to cope with the actual disease and prevent its further transmission.

Volumes have been written about the treatment of HIV/AIDS; new information appears in the electronic or print media daily. *HIV/AIDS Nursing Secrets* is a concise reference for experienced and novice nurses working with clients who have HIV/AIDS. It is also relevant for other health care professionals and lay persons interested in HIV/AIDS because of the broad nature of the content, clarity of presentation, and glossary for easy identification of terms. The content focuses on providing the holistic, clinically competent care that all clients require.

The book is organized into four parts to help the reader understand the multiple facets of HIV/AIDS care: origins, epidemiology, pathophysiology, and nursing interventions; conditions that compound the problems of dealing with HIV/AIDS; vulnerable populations; and cultures and subcultures. Sources of additional information about various topics, especially websites, are included in the chapters.

We sincerely appreciate the knowledge, expertise, commitment, and diversity of our contributors. Chapter authors represent varied areas of clinical practice, education, administration, and research as well as a varied geographic distribution. We also thank family and friends, especially Meg Shaw-Phalen, for their support and understanding during the completion of this work. Special thanks are given to Linda J. Scheetz, EdD, RN, CS, CEN, for asking us to create this necessary addition to the Nursing Secrets Series®.

Judy K. Shaw, MS, ACRN, ANP-C
Elizabeth Anne Mahoney, RN, MSN, EdD, ACRN

I. HIV/AIDS: Origins and Trends

1. EPIDEMIOLOGY OF HIV

Christine Johnsen, MPH, RN, CS

Since human immunodeficiency virus (HIV) disease was first recognized over 20 years ago, much has been learned about its epidemiology and treatment. In high-income countries, with the availability of effective but costly medications, HIV infection and acquired immunodeficiency syndrome (AIDS) have evolved from a fatal illness to a chronic disease. In resource-poor countries, on the other hand, HIV/AIDS continues to have a devastating effect on individuals, families, communities, and society at large as a result of high mortality rates, particularly in young people of reproductive age and their offspring.

1. Summarize the history of the HIV epidemic from the first reported cases.

The first recognized cases of AIDS were reported in the summer of 1981 in the United States. Young homosexual men were diagnosed with *Pneumocystis carinii* pneumonia (PCP) and Kaposi's sarcoma (KS), two diseases that were not previously seen in this population. In high-income countries, the next groups to manifest HIV disease were recipients of blood and blood products, then injection drug users, and finally infants of women exposed through injection drug use or sexual relations with injection drug users.

Although Europe and North America were the first to recognize an early epidemic of HIV, the major locus of the epidemic is in resource-poor countries. The recognition of HIV in resource-poor countries was delayed by the presence of an already heavy disease burden in these populations. A heterosexual AIDS epidemic was recognized in Africa in 1983, and by 1985 at least one case of HIV/AIDS had been reported in every region of the world.

2. How do the earliest projections of the AIDS epidemic to the year 2000 compare with the actual 2000 rates?

Since the HIV/AIDS epidemic was first identified over 20 years ago, its scale and severity have exceeded all expectations. In 1991, the World Health Organization (WHO) forecast a cumulative total of 40 million cases of HIV infection by the year 2000. An estimated 40 million people are living with HIV today, and 20 million have died—a cumulative total of 60 million people. It is expected that, given current rates of infection and the long lag between infection and development of symptoms, the most devastating impact is yet to come.

At the beginning of the twentieth century, infectious diseases were the leading cause of death worldwide. Infectious disease mortality rates declined in the United States and elsewhere in the developed world during the first eight decades of the twentieth century as a result of improvements in living conditions, sanitation, medical care, and public health programs; rates declined further with the introduction of antibiotics and mass immunization programs. Infectious diseases have remained leading causes of death in the developing world, and, at the end of the twentieth century, infectious disease mortality is increasing in the developed world as well. Factors that have influenced the re-emergence of infectious diseases include changes in human behavior, technology, and the environment; development of drug-resistant pathogens; and newly recognized microorganisms, including HIV.

The successful spread of HIV has occurred for many reasons. The discovery of penicillin and other antibiotics has led to the treatment and cure of most sexually transmitted diseases

1

(STDs). Antibiotics and hormonal contraceptives for birth control have resulted in changes in sexual practices, including unprotected sex and multiple sexual partners. The concomitant use of drugs and alcohol is associated with increased high-risk sexual behavior. In Africa, the rapid spread of HIV among heterosexual populations has been facilitated by social and economic factors. The building of roads allows long-distance travel, social migration, and sexual mixing. International travel has converted the world into a global village, facilitating the spread of diseases transmitted by person-to-person contact.

3. What is the status of the global HIV/AIDS epidemic at the beginning of the twenty-first century?

An estimated 40 million people currently live with HIV/AIDS worldwide. Of 37.2 million adults with HIV/AIDS worldwide, 48% are women. Approximately one-third of those living with HIV/AIDS are young people between 15 and 24 years of age; most of them do not know that they are infected. There are 2.7 million children under 15 years of age with HIV/AIDS worldwide. In 2001, an estimated 5 million people were newly infected with HIV, including 800,000 children. There were 3 million AIDS-related deaths in 2001, including 580,000 children. HIV/AIDS is the fourth leading cause of death in the world. Global trends in HIV/AIDS are presented in the table on the facing page.

4. Describe the prevalence and incidence in Sub-Saharan Africa.

Sub-Saharan Africa is the most affected region in the world, with 70% of the world's HIV/AIDS population. There were approximately 3.4 million new infections in 2001, bringing the total number of people living with HIV/AIDS in this region to 28.1 million. Women account for 55% of adult cases, the highest proportion of women with HIV in any region of the world. AIDS is the leading cause of death in Sub-Saharan Africa. Of the 1.1 million children with HIV, over 90% were infected through mother-infant transmission. Sixteen countries make up the Sub-Saharan region, where the average infection rate is 8.8% in adults. Botswana has the highest prevalence, with 36% of adults infected with HIV.

A report by the United Nations AIDS (UNAIDS) program predicts that as many as one-half of adolescents in some southern African countries will die from AIDS, including two-thirds of 15-year-olds in Botswana.[14] Demographers predict that in any country where 15% of adults are now infected, at least 35% of adolescents will eventually die of AIDS.

In general, the HIV epidemic in Sub-Saharan Africa is fueled by poverty, inequality, and migration, generated largely by heterosexual transmission with significant mother-infant transmission. The HIV prevalence among pregnant women attending antenatal clinics in South Africa was < 1% in 1990; yet by the end of 2000, the prevalence among pregnant South African women increased to 24.5%. In some countries (e.g., Zambia, Uganda), effective prevention measures have resulted in a decrease in the prevalence among young people, particularly women, and a reduction in the rate of perinatal transmission.

At the end of 2001, more than 10 African countries were providing antiretroviral therapy to people living with HIV/AIDS. Education and condom distribution programs are resulting in increased awareness and condom usage, reports of fewer multiple partners, and declining prevalence among urban residents in some areas. Yet the vast majority of HIV-infected Africans still do not know that they are infected.

5. What are the prevalence and incidence in Asia and the Pacific Islands?

The epidemic in Asia and the Pacific Islands started in the late 1980s; now about 7.1 million people are infected. An estimated 1.07 million new infections in Asia and the Pacific Islands were reported in 2001. The epidemic is driven by injection drug use, heterosexual transmission, and unprotected sex between men. An estimated 35% of infected adults in Asia and 20% of infected adults in the Pacific Islands are women.

The HIV epidemic in this region is linked closely to the epidemic in injection drug use. Recent observations in China suggest dramatic increases in this population. Sentinel surveillance

Regional HIV/AIDS Statistics and Features, End of 2001

REGION	EPIDEMIC STARTED	PEOPLE LIVING WITH HIV/AIDS	PEOPLE NEWLY INFECTED	ADULT PREVALENCE RATE*	% INFECTED ADULTS WHO ARE WOMEN	MAIN MODE OF TRANSMISSION FOR ADULTS
Sub-Saharan Africa	Late 1970s Early 1980s	28.1 million	3.4 million	8.4%	55%	Heterosexual activity
North Africa and Middle East	Late 1980s	440,000	80,000	0.2%	40%	Heterosexual activity, injection drug use
South and Southeast Asia	Late 1980s	6.1 million	800,000	0.6%	35%	Heterosexual activity, injection drug use
East Asia and Pacific Islands	Late 1980s	1 million	270,000	0.1%	20%	Injection drug use, heterosexual activity men who have sex with men
Latin America	Late 1970s Early 1980s	1.4 million	130,000	0.5%	30%	Men who have sex with men, injection drug use, heterosexual activity
Caribbean Islands	Late 1970s Early 1980s	420,000	60,000	2.2%	50%	Heterosexual activity, men who have sex with men
Eastern Europe and Central Asia	Early 1990s	1 million	250,000	0.5%	20%	Injection drug use
Western Europe	Late 1970s Early 1980s	560,000	30,000	0.3%	25%	Men who have sex with men, injection drug use
North America	Late 1970s Early 1980s	940,000	45,000	0.6%	20%	Men who have sex with men, injection drug use, heterosexual activity
Australia and New Zealand	Late 1970s Early 1980s	15,000	500	0.1%	10%	Men who have sex with men
Totals		40 million	5 million	1.2%	48%	

* The proportion of adults (15–49 years of age) living with HIV/AIDS in 2001, using 2001 population numbers.
From AIDS Epidemic Update. December 2001 UNAIDS/WHO 2001. UNAIDS/01.74E-WHO/CDS/CSR/ NCS/2001.

among injection drug users detected no HIV infection in 1995 at eight surveillance sites, but in 1998 detected HIV in 17 of 19 sites. The highest prevalence among injection drug users was 82% in Yining City in the western Xinjiang province. Serious epidemics have occurred in Central China as a result of improper blood-processing procedures for transfusions. HIV prevalence rates up to 6% have been observed in sex workers, and rates of STDS have risen dramatically, indicating the potential for HIV spread in the future.

Elsewhere in this region, the epidemic is quite diverse. In India, with a population of 1 billion, an estimated 3.9 million people are infected. In Indonesia, after a decade of negligible rates, prevalence has increased recently in sex workers and injection drug users. The prevalence of infection in injection drug users is 40% in Jakarta and > 50% in Bali, Myanmar, Nepal, Thailand, and Manipur (in India). Prevention programs can and do work in this region. Thailand's comprehensive prevention program has reduced the number of new infections from a high of 140,000/year a decade ago to 30,000/year recently.

6. What about Eastern Europe and Central Asia?

HIV incidence is increasing at the fastest rate in this region of the world. The epidemic started here in the early 1990s. There were an estimated 250,000 new cases in 2001, bringing the total number of cases to 1 million. The epidemic is confined mostly to injection dug users, but the proportion of sexually transmitted HIV infections is increasing. An estimated 20% of all adult cases are in women; however, the female-to-male ratio among new cases of HIV is 1:2, indicating an increased risk of infection among young women in this region.

7. Describe the prevalence and incidence in Latin America and the Caribbean.

An estimated 1.8 million people live with HIV in this region, including 190,000 newly infected people. With an average prevalence of 2%, the Caribbean is the second most affected region in the world; 50% of adult cases are in women. The epidemic started in the late 1970s, and, taken as a whole, the incidence is not increasing. Rates are increasing in several Central American countries, mostly as a result of heterosexual transmission. In Haiti by the end of 1999, the prevalence rate among the adult population exceeded 5%, the highest rate outside Africa. In Brazil, however, incidence rates are low, and a substantial decline in HIV prevalence in injection drug users has been observed as a result of strong prevention efforts and wide access to antiretroviral therapy.

8. How are high-income countries affected?

In Western Europe, North America, Australia, and New Zealand, an estimated 1.5 million people live with HIV/AIDS. The epidemic started in the late 1970s. The adult prevalence rate is < 1%, and 20–25% of adult cases are women. Men who have sex with men continue to be the main transmission route. HIV is moving into poor communities, with women and people of color at particular risk. Prevalence has also increased in high-income countries because of increased survival as a result of access to antiretroviral therapy.

In Japan, HIV infection is increasing among men who have sex with men. Evidence indicates that the sexual behavior of Japan's youth is placing them at higher risk of HIV, with increasing rates of sexually transmitted disease and low condom use.

9. What is the status of the HIV/AIDS epidemic in the United States?

At the end of December 2000, the Centers for Disease Control and Prevention (CDC) reported 774,467 cumulative cases of AIDS in the United States since 1981. Nearly 99% of these cumulative cases were persons 13 years of age or older, and 82% were male. Male-to-male sex has been the most common mode of exposure, accounting for 46% of cases, followed by injection drug use (25% of cases) and heterosexual contact (11%).

10. How many people are living with HIV/AIDS in the U.S.?

Through December 2000, 450,151 people had been reported to the CDC as living with HIV/AIDS: 127,058 with HIV and 312,946 with AIDS. In 2001, the CDC estimates the number of people living with HIV or AIDS in the U.S. at 800,000–900,000. The estimated number is almost double the reported number of cases of HIV/AIDS for several reasons: not all states report HIV infection, many people obtain anonymous tests, and not everyone is aware of his or her HIV status.

11. How many people are newly diagnosed with AIDS in the U.S.?
In the year 2000, there were 42,156 newly reported cases of AIDS in the United States, and 99.5% involved people aged 13 years or older. Of these, 47% were black and 19% were Hispanic. Of the 196 children newly diagnosed with AIDS in 2000, 65% were black and 17% were Hispanic. Ninety percent of these children were infected perinatally.

In 1999, the predominant mode of HIV exposure among an estimated 31,590 adult and adolescent men diagnosed with AIDS was male-to-male sex (53%). The predominant mode of exposure among an estimated 10,092 adult and adolescent women diagnosed with AIDS in 1999 was heterosexual contact.

12. How many people are newly diagnosed with HIV in the U.S.?
In 2000, 21,704 newly diagnosed cases of HIV (not AIDS) were reported from 36 areas: 68% were adult men, 31% were adult women, and 1% were children under 13 years of age. The CDC estimates that approximately 40,000 new HIV infections occur in the US every year and that 70% of these new HIV infections occur among men. By risk, men who have sex with men represent the largest group of new infections (42%), followed by men and women who are exposed through heterosexual activity (33%) and injection drug use (25%). By race, 54% of new HIV infections occur among blacks, although they represent only 13% of the U.S. population. Hispanics account for 19% of new HIV infections and only 12% of the U.S. population.

13. How many people have died from AIDS in the U.S.?
The total number of deaths attributed to AIDS is 448,060, including 442,882 adults and adolescents and 5,178 children under age 13. In 2000, 8,867 AIDS-related deaths occurred in adults and adolescents, and 44 deaths were reported in children under 13 years of age. Data from the CDC[7] indicate a dramatic decline in AIDS deaths among adults and adolescents with the introduction of highly active antiretroviral therapy in the mid 1990s. The estimated death rate declined by 42% from 1996 to 1997, but only by 8% from 1998 to 1999. The leveling of deaths may reflect a slowing of the decline in AIDS incidence as well as limitations of current therapies in treatment-experienced populations.

14. Discuss the geographic distribution of HIV/AIDS in the U.S.
Fifty-four percent of the estimated 317,652 people living with AIDS in 1999 lived in five states: New York (17%), California (14%), Florida (11%), Texas (7%), and New Jersey (5%). Over 40% of people with AIDS lived in 10 cities, with the greatest numbers in Los Angeles, New York City, and Washington, D.C. By region, 119,430 or nearly 38% of people with AIDS in 1999 lived in the South; 95,445 or 30% lived in the Northeast; 62,357 or 20% lived in the West; and nearly 10% lived in the Midwest.

15. How have children been exposed to HIV in the U.S.?
Since the beginning of the AIDS epidemic, a total of 8,908 cases of AIDS has been reported among children under age 13. The majority of these children (91%) were exposed perinatally, nearly 3% had hemophilia or other coagulation disorders, and 4% were other recipients of infected blood or tissue. Nearly all transmission of HIV through blood or blood products occurred before 1985, when screening of the blood supply for HIV was initiated. Currently, in the U.S. and globally, the majority of children were exposed perinatally.

16. What are the trends in the perinatal HIV epidemic?
Vertical or perinatal transmission occurs during pregnancy, labor, and delivery and through breastmilk. Without intervention, the transmission rate in high-income countries is 14–25% and up to 40–45% in resource-poor countries.

An estimated 2.7 million children worldwide live with HIV, and over 90% were infected perinatally. Sixteen hundred infants are born with HIV every day in the world. There are two perinatal epidemics. In high-income countries with well-established health infrastructures that provide HIV counseling and testing, antiretroviral therapy, surgical obstetric practices, and infant formula in lieu of breastmilk, vertical HIV transmission can be reduced to < 2% by using all available interventions. In contrast, resource-poor countries, with scant or no health infrastructures, have a limited ability to conduct HIV counseling and testing, limited availability of antiretroviral therapy, and no alternative to breastmilk; thus, they experience high perinatal transmission rates of 40–45%.

During the early 1990s, an estimated 1,000–2,000 infants were born with HIV infection each year in the U.S. In 1994, the Pediatric AIDS Clinical Trials Group (PACTG) 07613 demonstrated the benefit of a three-part regimen of zidovudine (ZVD) monotherapy: orally to mothers during their pregnancy, intravenously to mothers during labor and delivery, and to infants for the first 6 weeks of life. Transmission was reduced from 25% to 8% in the ZVD-treated group. Combination antiretroviral therapy with protease inhibitors, an elective cesarean delivery, and the avoidance of breastfeeding can reduce transmission to < 2%. Since the PACTG report, perinatal transmission has dropped dramatically. In 1999, 263 cases of pediatric AIDS were reported, most of whom were infected perinatally. Over 90% of HIV-infected mothers and/or their infants in the U.S. received ZVD in 1999.

An estimated 20% of perinatal transmission occurs in utero as evidenced by the detection of HIV in aborted fetuses and the benefit of earlier vs. later intervention during pregnancy. Eighty percent of transmission is thought to occur late in pregnancy, especially during labor and delivery through exposure to infected blood and secretions, as evidenced by the increased risk of firstborn twins, prolonged labor or prolonged rupture of membranes, and the benefits of elective cesarean delivery and a single dose of an antiretroviral medication administered to the mother during labor and then to the infant.

17. What are the gender differences globally and in the United States?

Nearly 50% of people infected with HIV worldwide are women. In many countries, even if women know how to protect themselves, lack of access to condoms and lack of sexual autonomy prevent them from doing so. The high rates of HIV among women in resource-poor countries and among poor and minority women in high-income countries reflect the vulnerability of women as a result of limited access to information about HIV transmission and prevention, medical care for treatment of STDs and HIV, and inability to negotiate sexual safety.

Gender equality is an essential element in the fight against AIDS. In Africa, as in many other countries, women lack control over their bodies, are vulnerable to dispossession by their husbands, have low literacy levels, and have little access to paid employment outside the home, except for commercial sex work. Sexual practices such as genital mutilation, "dry sex," the mythical cure of HIV by having sex with a virgin, and rape, including marital rape, increase a woman's risk of HIV infection. Increased awareness of gender-based injustice and a change in women's social status are needed to empower women to protect themselves.

18. Why do 95% of the estimated 40 million people infected with HIV live in the developing world?

HIV is spread mostly by sexual contact and injection drug use. HIV travels along the routes of human movement: migration of labor forces, trucking, drug trafficking, and migration as a result of war. Transmission is facilitated by lack of knowledge, presence of sexually transmitted disease, and the low status of women and adolescents.

The pattern of the African epidemic matches migrant labor patterns. Colvin and Sharp's study in South Africa[12] indicated that all cases of HIV in villages occurred along the main road. Another study[11] reported that the HIV prevalence among factory workers who lived apart from their wives was 13.7% compared with 0% among workers who stayed at home.

In Southeast Asia the escalation of the HIV epidemic is associated with commercial sex workers and injection drug use. Urban sex workers in Thailand, Burma, Cambodia, and India have HIV infection rates between 20% and 60%. In Eastern Europe, an estimated fivefold increase in HIV in the late 1990s is believed to be a result of injection drug use.

In the past two decades the globalization of capital has resulted in increased urbanization, a decline in rural subsistence economies, increased rural poverty, increased migration for work, and an increase in trucking. As a result of these changing economies, there has been an increase in unemployment, especially for women, forcing many into commercial sex work. Reduced funds for health and education have left many countries without an adequate health infrastructure for STD treatment and HIV prevention programs.

Finally, the global economy has resulted in increased liberalization of capital transactions, allowing not only legal but also illegal transfers of huge sums of money, such as money from illegal drug transactions, fostering a prosperous illicit drug trade.

19. Have effective interventions been identified?

Effective interventions are available. Generally, however, successful programs require strong high-level political leadership, a national plan, strong community involvement, and adequate funding that has not been available. Quality testing and guidelines for blood use can promote a safer blood supply. Widespread condom promotion can reduce transmission in high-risk populations. Sex education programs can decrease risk-taking behaviors in young people. Substance abuse treatment and harm reduction programs can reduce the risk of infection in illicit drug-using populations. Improved STD treatment can slow HIV infection rates.

Many young people in developing countries are unaware of how the virus is transmitted and how they can protect themselves from infection. In many countries, even if women know how to protect themselves, their lack of access to condoms and lack of sexual autonomy prevent them from doing so.

Prevention and treatment are the most effective interventions. Treatments that reduce both horizontal and perinatal transmission have been dramatically effective in reducing mother-to-child transmission. Treatment improves quality of life and reduces morbidity and mortality rates. Treatment offers hope. The United Nations Secretary-General has called for a global health fund to integrate the prevention, treatment, and care of HIV, tuberculosis, and malaria, the three leading causes of death worldwide.

BIBLIOGRAPHY

1. Armstrong GL, Conn LA, Pinner RW: Trends in infectious disease mortality in the United States during the 20th century. JAMA 281: 61–66, 1999.
2. Anderson J, ed: A Guide to the Clinical Care of Women with HIV. Washington, DC, HRSA and HIV/AIDS Bureau, 2000.
3. Berkman A: Confronting global AIDS: Prevention and treatment. Am J Public Health 91:1348–1349, 2001.
4. Centers for Disease Control and Prevention: HIV/AIDS surveillance report 12 (No. 2):1–48, 2000
5. Centers for Disease Control and Prevention: HIV/AIDS surveillance supplemental report (No. 1):1–16, 2001.
6. Centers for Disease Control and Prevention: First report of AIDS. MMWR 50:429, 2001.
7. Centers for Disease Control and Prevention: HIV/AIDS—United States, 1981–2000. MMWR 50:430–434, 2001.
8. Centers for Disease Control and Prevention: The global HIV/AIDS epidemic, 2001. MMWR 50:434–439, 2001.
9. Centers for Disease Control and Prevention: HIV/AIDS Update. www.cdc.gov/hiv/pubs/facts.htm (accessed 26 Dec 2001).
10. Cohen ML: Changing patterns of infectious diseases. Nature 406:762–767, 2000.
11. Colvin M, et al: HIV infection and asymptomatic sexually transmitted infections in a rural South African community. Int J STD AIDS 9:548–550, 1998.
12. Colvin M, Sharp B: Sexually transmitted infections and HIV in a rural community in the Lesotho highlands. Sex Transm Infect 76 (1):39–42, 2000.
13. Connor EM, et al: Reduction of maternal-infant transmission of human immunodeficiency virus type 1 with zidovudine treatment. N Engl J Med 331:1173–1180, 1994.

14. Gottlieb S: UN says up to half the teenagers in Africa will die of AIDS. Br Med J 321:67, 2000.
15. Karon JM, et al: HIV in the United States at the turn of the century: An epidemic in transition. Am J Public Health 91:1060–1068, 2001.
16. Kline M, et al: Technical report: Perinatal human immunodeficiency virus testing and prevention of transmission. Pediatrics 106:88, 2001.
17. Piot P, et al: The global impact of HIV/AIDS. Nature 410:968–973, 2001.
18. Rankin W, Wilson C: African women with HIV: Faith-based answers might ease the social problems that lead to AIDS. Br Med J 321:1543–1544, 2000.
19. Rosenfield A: After Cairo: Women's reproductive and sexual health, rights and empowerment. Am J Public Health 90:1838–1840, 2000.
20. Shahmanesh M, et al: AIDS and globalization. Sex Transm Infect 76:154–155, 2000.
21. UNAIDS: The global strategy framework on HIV/AIDS. June 2001. www.unaids.org/publications/documents/care/general/JC637-GlobalFramew-E.pdf (accessed 8 Jan 02).
22. UNAIDS/WHO: 20 years of HIV/AIDS. June 2001. UNAIDS/WHO 2001. www.unaids.org/UNGASS/index.html (accessed 8 Jan 02).
23. UNAIDS/WHO: Children and young people in a world of AIDS. August 2001. UNAIDS/WHO 2001. www.unaids.org/publications/documents/children/children/JC656-child&AIDS-E.pdf (accessed 8 Jan 02).
24. UNAIDS/WHO: AIDS Epidemic Update. December 2001. UNAIDS/WHO 2001. (UNAIDS/01.74E-WHO/CDS/CSR/NCS/2001.2) www.unaids.org/epidemic-ypdate/report_dec01/index.html (accessed 8 Jan 02).

2. WHAT IS GOING ON INSIDE?

Vi Wilkes, MS, MA, ACRN

The discussion of what is going on inside touches on central issues such as characteristics of the human immunodeficiency virus (HIV), how it infects humans, how it damages the immune system, how it is diagnosed, the rationale of treatment, and the prognosis.

1. What is HIV?

HIV is a virus that attacks and destroys the cells of the immune system. Untreated, the person infected with HIV becomes progressively susceptible to life-threatening viruses and bacteria. Finally, the person with terminal HIV disease dies because the immune system is destroyed and can no longer mount a defense against even common bacterial and viral invasions.

2. How did HIV infect humans?

There are various beliefs about the origin of HIV. Many experts think that the virus originated in West Africa and may have emerged after it crossed the host-species barrier from the African green monkey to humans. The rationale for this thinking is the striking similarity between HIV and the simian immunodeficiency virus (SIV). The African monkey carries SIV without clinical disease presentation. Other experts speculate that HIV crossed the host-species barrier when scientists and researchers compounded the Salk polio vaccine with African green monkey serum and tested the vaccine on African children in the mid and late 1950s.

3. How did HIV appear in the United States?

HIV appeared in the United States in 1981[5] with the report of five cases of *Pneumocystis carinii* pneumonia in Los Angeles. The common thread was that the men were white, young, and homosexual. Similar cases emerged in New York. Because HIV occurred in gay populations, there was a general lack of concern on the part of the public and public officials. The emergence of HIV in United States occurred against the backdrop of homophobia, ignorance, apathy, political and bureaucratic red tape, and downright negligence. Finally, as the disease appeared in other populations, such as persons of Haitian origin and people with IV drug addiction, hemophilia, sickle cell disease, and renal failure, attention turned toward the search for a causative agent

4. When did the HIV antibody test appear?

Sande and Volberding[12] reported that the technology for the HIV antibody test was available before the HIV virus was isolated in 1983. However, it was not until 1985 that the test for the HIV antibody was used routinely to screen blood and blood products and to test people at risk for HIV infection. Before the nation's blood supply was tested for HIV, HIV-tainted blood and blood products were freely administered and became the cause of many HIV infections in people receiving blood for hemophilia, renal failure, trauma, and surgery.

5. How is HIV transmitted?

HIV targets the white blood cells, specifically the T4 cells. Therefore, HIV is acquired by contact with bodily fluids containing white cells, including blood and semen. Modes of transmission include oral, vaginal, and anal sexual intercourse with partners infected with HIV, IV drug use with infected needles, infusion of tainted blood, perinatal transmission, and occupational exposure.

6. What are the crucial characteristics of HIV?

The crucial characteristics of HIV include virology, taxonomy, genome, subtypes, life cycle, epidemiology, effects on the immune system, manifestations of acute or primary infection, and the Centers for Disease Control and Prevention (CDC) classification of HIV infection.

7. What are the major subtypes of HIV?

There are two major subtypes of HIV. HIV-I, which is most prevalent in the United States, is often considered by experts as more acute, virulent, and progressive. HIV-II is found in Africa, Haiti, and other third-world countries.

8. How is HIV classified?

HIV belongs to a family of retroviruses, which are so designated because during replication the viral ribonucleic acid (RNA) transcribes viral DNA by the action of the enzyme reverse transcriptase (RT). This process is a reversal of the norm, in which DNA transcribes RNA.

9. What properties do retroviruses have in common?

Retroviruses are enveloped in a capsule, have a cell membrane bud that attaches to the target cell, and are extracellular or outside the cellular compartment. The modes of transmission can be endogenous and are similar to those of the human T-cell lymphotrophic virus (HTLV), which may be inherited vertically. Alternatively, the retroviruses can be transmitted through direct contact with infected blood and body fluids.

All of the retroviruses have three genes in common that code for (1) the internal viral core protein (*gag* gene), (2) reverse transcriptase (*pol* gene), and (3) the outer viral envelope protein (*env* gene). These three viral genes are involved in viral replication. The viruses have an outer envelop with eccentric buds projecting from the cell membrane. The viruses are designed to attach to the target cell membrane, shed the outer coat once inside the target cell, transcribe (via reverse transcriptase) viral RNA into proviral DNA, insert the proviral DNA into the cell's DNA, and then use the target cell's nutrients and energy to replicate. The genes are identified by their protein or glycoprotein composition and are measured by molecular weight in Daltons.

Properties of Retroviruses

PROPERTY	MODES OF TRANSMISSION	REPLICATION	GENES IN COMMON
Envelope	Endogenous	Inherited*	Internal core protein
Cell membrane bud	Exogenous	Transmitted	Reverse transcriptase
Extracellular			Envelope glycoprotein

* Some strains of HTLV are exogenous and inherited vertically.

10. How was HIV discovered?

The discovery of HIV was surrounded by controversy. Robert Gallo, a researcher from the U.S. National Institute of Health, claimed the discovery. However, Luc Montagnier, a French researcher, claimed that the virus was originally isolated in the Pasteur Clinic in Paris and that he had loaned the virus to Gallo. The two researchers are credited equally with the discovery of HIV.

HIV was originally identified as HTLV-III because HIV was structurally similar to HTLV-I and HTLV-II. HTLV targets the lymphocytes, specifically the T cells. According to Sande and Volberding,[12] the HTLV-III virus was renamed human immunodeficiency virus (HIV) by an international taxonomy committee in 1986. The HIV genome is similar in molecular structure to the genomes of HTLV-I, which causes T-cell leukemia and T-cell lymphoma, and HTLV-II.

Human Retroviruses and Clinical Presentation*

VIRUS	CLINICAL PRESENTATION
HTLV-I	Adult T-cell leukemia/lymphoma
HTLV-II	Unknown
HIV-I (HTLV-III)	HIV infection and AIDS
HIV-II (HTLV-IV)	HIV infection and AIDS found in Africa
Spumavirus	Not associated with disease

* Retroviruses affecting animals are not shown.

11. How are retroviruses further classified?

Retroviruses can be classified into two subtypes: lentiviruses and oncoviruses. HIV is classified as a lentivirus. Lentiviruses are so named because *lenti* means slow and the viruses in this family have a long incubation period, sometimes taking years to replicate and present clinically in infected persons. HIV is known to have a long latency period characterized by few or no symptoms, followed by viral activation, progression, and chronic illness. Alternatively, the virus can be virulent and aggressive, quickly progressing from seroconversion to full-blown AIDS.

Subtypes of Human Retroviruses

LENTIVIRUSES	ONCOVIRUSES
HIV-I,	HTLV-I,
HIV-II	HTLV-II
	Spumavirus

12. What does HIV look like? How is the genome organized?

The virus is round and has two coats or envelopes. The genes *gp 120* and *gp 41* (*env*) code for the outer and inner coatings, respectively. Three *gag* proteins, *p15*, *p17*, and *p24*, code for the viral core. The gene *p66* (*pol*) codes for reverse transcriptase, the enzyme that transcribes viral RNA into proviral DNA. The proviral DNA is then integrated (through the enzyme integrase) into the DNA of host cells. The genes code for a virus that is designed to outsmart the immune system. The virus mutates into different strains and selectively changes the way that the genes are expressed, making the development of a vaccine against the virus a difficult task.

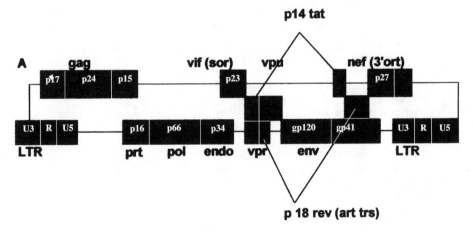

HIV genome organization. (Adapted from Beshe R: Genome organization of human immunodeficiency virus. In Beshe R (ed): Textbook of Human Virology, 2nd ed. St. Louis, Mosby, 1991, p 277, with permission.)

13. What do the other genes do?

The other genes code for the following functions:
- *LTR* (long terminal repeats): controls replication.
- *tat*: thought to be the master gene of replication.
- *rev*: selectively regulates synthesis of structural genes (*pol*, *env*, and *gag*).
- *nef*: a negative factor that downregulates replication.
- *vif*: controls infectivity.
- *vpr*: arrests cell cycle and influences progression.
- *vpu*: destroys CD4 cells on viral budding and also influences gene progression.

14. What is the significance of the life cycle of the HIV?

HIV primarily targets and attacks the T4 cell. The virus enters the cell and either remains latent or multiplies. If the virus multiplies, the CD4 cell is often destroyed.

Binding
HIV gp 120 seeks out the T4 cell and binds to its CD4 receptor
↓

Uncoating
Inside the T4 cell, the virus sheds its two outer coats, releasing two copies of RNA
↓

Transcription
Viral RNA is transcribed by RT (p66, *pol*) into proviral DNA
↓

Integration
Proviral DNA is integrated into the T4 DNA by the enzyme integrase (p34)
↓

Translation
mRNA (that includes HIV genetic material) is produced by the T4 cell for cell division
↓

Assembly
Via RNA Polymerase II, the HIV core, envelop, and RT are assembled
↓

Budding and Maturation
The new HIV buds from the T4 cell and matures with the assistance of HIV protease (p16)

Life cycle of the human immunodeficiency virus. (This figure was based on readings in Belshe,[3] Kuby,[8] McDonald and Kuritzkes,[9] and Sande and Volberding[12]).

15. What drugs are currently used or could be used to block the action of each step in the life cycle of HIV?

Pharmacologic treatment is often directed toward blocking one of the steps in the life cycle of HIV (see Chapter 4). Treatment of HIV includes drugs that:
- Prevent binding to stop HIV from fusing to the CD4 receptor of the T4 cell.
- Block the action of reverse transcriptase (e.g., azidothymidine and the nonnucleoside analogs) to prevent HIV RNA from transcribing to DNA, thereby preventing new virons from forming.
- Block integrase (integrase antagonists), thus preventing the integration of viral DNA into the T4 cell DNA.
- Block translation, which may prevent mRNA translation and formation of a new viron.
- Block the maturation of a new viron, similar to the action of the protease inhibitors. In this case, the virus is assembled and released but is immature and unable to infect other T4 cells.

16. What happens in the body when HIV attacks?

HIV targets and attacks the white blood cells. Although it is now known that HIV targets other white cells, the T4 cell with its CD4 (cell-differentiated) receptor is the primary target for HIV. The table at the top of the following page shows the differentiation of the white blood cells. The lymphocytes provide cell-mediated (T cells) and humoral immunity (B cells) for the body. The T cells have regulator and effector functions. T4 cells also may be called CD4s because of the CD4 receptors attached to their outer membrane. HIV has a receptor bud on the cell surface that is designed as an exact match for the receptor on the T4 cell's membrane surface. The two receptors attach and fuse while HIV inserts its deadly contents into the T4 cell.

17. How do the T cells regulate the immune system?

When a viral threat presents, the T cells mount an immune response with the helper T cells (T4s). The T cells are the master cells of the immune system. They monitor the immune response and stimulate the production of more T cells, B cells, and lymphokines. The T cells also know when a virus is defeated and send suppressor T cells (T8s) to turn off the immune response. There is some speculation, however, that the overabundance of suppressor T8s may actually enhance the ability of HIV to gain entrance into cells.[12]

18. How do the T cells carry out the cytotoxic function?

The T cells produce lymphokines that are toxic to viruses and some tumors. In addition, T cells have the ability to destroy viruses directly through their own cytotoxicity and the cytotoxicity of natural killer cells. Antigen-presenting cells display a piece of the antigen (in this case, HIV) on their surface for other cells in the immune system to see and destroy.

19. How do the B cells convey humoral immunity?

The B cells provide humoral immunity by making antibodies against invading viruses and other organisms. The antibodies are effective in destroying some of the virus. Antibodies to HIV are thought to kill free virus in the serum. However, once inside the T cells, the virus is safely tucked away from the watchful B cells. B cells also produce a mature plasma cell that stands ready for an invading organism and a memory cell that remembers an organism once it has been presented. The memory cell helps to mount an immune response more quickly against a returning invader.

*White Blood Cell Differentiation**

CELL TYPE	NORMAL MM³	NORMAL %	FUNCTION
Leukocytes	5–10,000		First line of defense against bacterial infection
Neutrophils			
Basophils			
Eosinophils			
Monocytes			
Lymphocytes	1500–4500		Cell-mediated (T cells) and humoral immunity (B cells)
T cells	900–1800	60–80	
T4	600–1100		
T8	450–600		
B cells	150–800	10–20	

* Values and percents are approximate.

20. Describe the natural history of HIV infection.

When a person has acquired HIV, the virus receptors have fused to the CD4 receptor of the T4 cell and implanted genetic materials inside the T4 cells. The virus may remain latent inside the T4 cell or replicate rapidly. Latent periods are known to last for as long as 10 years. If the virus begins to replicate, acute symptomatic HIV infection develops, and the person experiences symptoms similar to those caused by influenza. The incubation period can be 2–4 weeks.[12] Other symptoms may include lymphadenopathy, skin rashes, and ulcerations of the mucous membranes of the mouth, rectum, vagina, and penis.

21. What are the laboratory findings?

Laboratory studies show marked decreases in both CD4s and CD8s. The normal ratio of CD4 to CD8 is reversed, with the CD8 count greater than the CD4 count. While the CD4 count is decreasing, the p24 antigen (or the viral load) and the serum antibody to HIV are increasing. Characteristic laboratory results show a decrease in the lymphocyte count, a decrease in the T4 and T8 screens, an inverted T4/T8 ratio, and a decrease in red blood cell count and platelets. The table on the following page shows the laboratory results of a patient with progressive HIV infection who came to a clinic because of feeling "fatigued" and "not up to par." The patient reported having been infected about 5 years before but had never experienced symptoms or been treated.

Complete Blood Count with WBC Differential of a Patient with HIV Infection

TEST	VALUE[1000]	MEASURE UNIT	NORMAL
Red blood cell (RBC) count	3.70	mm^3	4.2–6.2
Hemoglobin	12.0	gm/dl	14.0–18.0
Hematocrit	34.6	%	41.0–52.0
White blood cell (WBC) count	3.3	mm^3	4.8–10.8
Neutrophils	80.0	%	40.0–70.0
Monocytes	8.0	%	2.0–8.0
Lymphocytes	10.0	%	20.0–45.0
T8	66.0	%	10.0–20.0
T4	13.1	%	60.0–80.0

22. Shall we do the math?

The table in question 21 shows that the RBC count, hemoglobin, and hematocrit are slightly decreased, which is a typical profile for a patient in this stage of HIV infection. To determine the absolute T4 count, we have to calculate the absolute lymphocyte count, using the following equation:

WBC count (1000) × lymphocyte % = absolute lymphocyte count
3.3 (1000) × 10% = 330 absolute lymphocyte count

From the absolute lymphocyte count, we calculate the absolute T4 count as follows:

Absolute lymphocyte count × T4 % = absolute T4 count
330 absolute lymphocytes × 13.1 % = 43.2 absolute T4 cell count

In this case, the patient's total T4 count was only 43.2 cells. A normal count would be near 1000. This patient illustrates the latency of HIV. Most likely, the patient's HIV infection was activated by another infection, and the virus replicated rapidly, reducing the T4 count to 43.2 before an opportunistic infection could be contracted. Because of the low T4 count, the patient was highly susceptible to many opportunistic infections. Work-up and treatment plans were developed.

The neutrophil count was near normal, as revealed by the following equation:

3.3 WBC (1000) × 80% = 2640 absolute neutrophil count

We can speculate that the neutrophils were not affected.

23. How does the virus progress in the body?

The rate of progression of HIV in the body varies. Time from seroconversion to development of symptoms may be months or years. Progression depends on the strain of the virus and the parts of the HIV genome that are expressed. For example, how the genes *vpr* and *vpu* are expressed is thought to affect progression. Host factors may affect disease progression in HIV infection. For example, Barber et al.[2] found that disease progression was more rapid in people who had a specific allele on the lymphocyte vitamin D receptors. People with this genotype had a reduced response to the immune-modulating effects of vitamin D and, therefore, were more susceptible to disease-activating factors.

The figure at the top of the following page shows a gross representation of the progression of HIV infection if the disease was left untreated. As the virus (p24) levels peak, the CD4 count decreases because the virus has destroyed the T4 cells. At the same time, the B cells have been activated, and the antibodies to the envelope glycoprotein (gp120) elevate in the serum. At this early stage, the patient will have the influenza-like symptoms and lymphadenopathy. The immune system has mounted a substantial immune response, as shown by the drop in the viral p24 antigen levels and the increase in the CD4s. However, the CD4s never return to the pre-HIV levels.

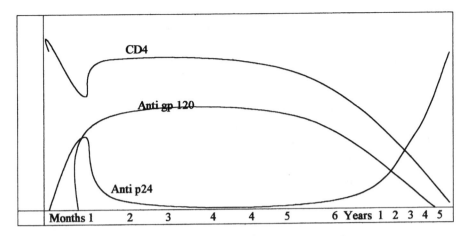

Progression of HIV infection and AIDS.

24. How long can the body keep HIV at bay?

The immune system is able to keep HIV under control for many months, as shown in the figure above. Even though HIV is produced, CD4 cells are also produced to destroy the virus. Because of the war between the immune system and the virus, the person with HIV infections experiences fever, fatigue, diarrhea, nausea, weight loss, headaches, and sometimes depression.

25. What happens when the immune system is no longer able to keep HIV in check?

The levels of the antibody to p24 antigen rise in the serum, CD4 levels decrease, and, for the first time, the antibody to gp120 decreases. The antibody decreases because the virus is also destroying this part of the immune system. The person with HIV infection in the terminal stages has a high viral load, anergy, and extreme immune deficiency. Death results from the opportunistic infections that take over in the absence of a competent immune system.

26. Explain the concept of efficiency as it applies to HIV.

The concept of efficiency of HIV refers to the capacity to infect per exposure. For example, receiving a unit of blood containing HIV produces an efficiency rate of 100% per unit of blood. Sexual intercourse with a person infected with the HIV has an efficiency rate of 0.1–1.0%, which means that the chance of acquiring the virus with one sexual act is 0.1–1.0%.

27. Explain the concept of infectivity.

Infectivity infers that the number of virons present in the serum alters the efficiency rates of transmission or acquisition of HIV. As demonstrated in the figure above, the viral load is higher during the acute and terminal stages of the infection. Kirtchner[7] established that higher levels of HIV in the serum were correlated with a higher rate of perinatal transmission. Pilcher et al.[11] found that sexual intercourse during the incubation period of HIV infection carried higher transmission rates because of the increased numbers of HIV in the blood. Transmission and acquisition of HIV are facilitated when the virus is present in the serum at higher levels.

28. How is HIV diagnosed?

The enzyme-linked immunosorbent assay (ELISA) detects IgG and IgM antibodies within approximately 6 weeks of the acute phase of infection. IgM antibody is evidence of a recent infection and is detected before IgG. Because of the window required for the body to make antibodies, the person can be HIV-positive and test negative. A positive ELISA is repeated and then confirmed by the Western Blot, which is more specific for antibodies against the HIV core and envelope proteins. The Western Blot uses a test strip that shows antibodies to three viral proteins. The presence of two or more on the test strip is considered a positive test for the HIV. The ELISA and the confirming Western Blot are the most frequently used tests for HIV detection and diagnosis.

According to the American Red Cross Website,[1] blood has been tested for HIV by the p24 antigen test since 1996. Before this time, blood was tested with the standard ELISA and confirmatory Western Blot. The p24 antigen, the viral core antigen, can be detected in the serum before seroconversion and sometimes within 24 hours of acute infection.[12] Other tests for HIV are used to monitor therapy rather than to diagnose HIV (see Chapter 4).

29. Summarize the CDC classification of AIDS.

In 1993 the CDC revised the criteria for classifying HIV infection and included CD4 categories in the staging system and case definition of AIDS. Thus, many people with HIV infection obtained an AIDS diagnosis, which assisted in documenting the need for medical disability and other financial assistance and benefits. The table below presents the CDC's 1993 revised classification system for HIV infection.[4]

People in category A have HIV infection with persistent granular lymphadenopathy or are asymptomatic; all have laboratory evidence of HIV infection. The subcategories of A1, A2, and A3 describe the clinical laboratory CD4 cell count in mm^3. As an example, an asymptomatic person with HIV infection and a CD4 count of 199 is classified as category A3, which is an AIDS-defining category.

Category B is similar to category A, except the person may have symptoms that are not related to the condition defined in category C of the CDC's 1993 AIDS surveillance case definition and does not fit into category A. Only B3 is an AIDS-defining category.

People who are classified in category C are considered to have AIDS. They have a low CD4 count and one of the opportunistic infections listed in category C.

The CDC Revised Classification System for HIV Infection, 1993*

CD4 CELLS (MM³)	CATEGORY A ASYMPTOMATIC ACUTE HIV OR PGL	CATEGORY B SYMPTOMATIC NOT A OR C	CATEGORY C INDICATOR CONDITIONS C IN AIDS SURVEILLANCE [†]
< 500	A1	B1	C1[‡]
200–499	A2	B2	C2[‡]
< 200	A3[‡]	B3[‡]	C3[‡]

PGL = persistent glandular lymphadenopathy.
* Based on information in MMWR 44(RR-17), 1993.
[†] Categories C1, C2, and C3 are AIDS-defining opportunistic diseases.
[‡] Categories A3, B3, C1, C2, and C3 are AIDS-defining categories.

30. Explain the significance of category B.

Conditions in category B must be a result of HIV infection; they take precedence over conditions in category A. The conditions are as follows:

- Bacillary angiomatosis
- Candidiasis, oropharyngeal (thrush)
- Candidiasis, vulvovaginal; persistent, frequent, or poorly responsive to therapy
- Cervical dysplasia (moderate or severe) or cervical carcinoma in situ
- Constitutional symptoms, such as fever (38.5°C) or diarrhea lasting longer than 1 month
- Hairy leukoplakia, oral
- Herpes zoster (shingles), involving at least two distinct episodes or more than one dermatome
- Idiopathic thrombocytopenic purpura
- Listeriosis
- Pelvic inflammatory disease, particularly if complicated by tubo-ovarian abscess
- Peripheral neuropathy[4]

31. Explain the significance of category C.

Category C is a repetition of conditions listed in the CDC's 1993 AIDS surveillance case definitions.[1] The AIDS surveillance case definition is a separate document that lists categories for how AIDS is defined and classified. The purpose of this case definition is to standardize reporting and statistical analyses that describe the causes of mortality and morbidity in people with AIDS. In addition, the categories are useful in monitoring people with HIV infection and AIDS and for documenting conditions for disability benefits. Category C conditions are as follows:

- Candidiasis of bronchi, trachea, or lungs
- Candidiasis, esophageal
- Cervical cancer, invasive
- Coccidioidomycosis, disseminated or extrapulmonary
- Cryptococcosis, extrapulmonary
- Cryptosporidiosis, chronic intestinal (more than 1 month's duration)
- Cytomegalovirus disease (other than liver, spleen, or nodes)
- Cytomegalovirus retinitis (with loss of vision)
- Encephalopathy, HIV-related
- Herpes simplex: chronic ulcer(s) (more than 1 month's duration) or bronchitis, pneumonitis, or esophagitis
- Histoplasmosis, disseminated or extrapulmonary
- Isosporiasis, chronic intestinal (more than 1 month's duration)
- Kaposi's sarcoma
- Lymphoma, Burkitt's (or equivalent term)
- Lymphoma, immunoblastic (or equivalent term)
- Lymphoma, primary, of brain
- *Mycobacterium avium* complex or *M. kansasii*, disseminated or extrapulmonary
- *Mycobacterium tuberculosis*, any site (pulmonary or extrapulmonary), or *Mycobacterium*, other or unidentified species, disseminated or extrapulmonary
- *Pneumocystis carinii* pneumonia
- Pneumonia, recurrent
- Progressive multifocal leukoencephalopathy
- *Salmonella* septicemia, recurrent
- Toxoplasmosis of brain
- Wasting syndrome due to HIV

32. What is the prognosis of HIV infection?

No cure currently exists for HIV infection and AIDS. The infection still results in mortality, even when treated. However, recent developments in testing and monitoring of viral load have led to improved diagnosis and treatment. In addition, the development, approval, and prescription of the protease inhibitors have rendered the virus undetectable in many persons with HIV infection who adhere to the treatment. Many resources are available: home kits for testing for HIV, an abundance of information about immune modulators and alternative therapy, and the ability to fine-tune pharmaceutical treatments. For example, drug combinations can be prescribed that take into account the resistance patterns of the virus specific to the person with HIV infection. HIV infection is now a chronic illness. Recent advances have added years to the lives of people living with HIV.

BIBLIOGRAPHY

1. American Red Cross Learning Center: How Blood is Tested. Available at http://www.pleasegive blood.org/learning/blood_testing.html.
2. Barber Y, Rubio C, Fernandez E, et al: Host genetic factors such as CCR5 chemokine receptors and vitamin D receptor loci and human immunodeficiency virus (HIV) type I disease among HIV-seropositive injection drug users. J Infect Dis 184:1279–1288, 2001.
3. Belshe R: Textbook of Human Virology, 2nd ed. St. Louis, Mosby, 1991.

4. Centers for Disease Control and Prevention: 1993 revised classification system for HIV infection and expanded surveillance case definition for AIDS among adolescents and adults. MMWR 44(RR-17), 1993. Available at http://www.cdc.gov/mmwr/preview/mmwrhtml/00018871.htm.

5. Centers for Disease Control and Prevention: First report of AIDS. MMWR 50 (20), 429, 2001. Available at http://www.cdc.gov/publications.

6. Centers for Disease Control and Prevention: HIV and AIDS—United States, 1981 to 2000. MMWR 50(21):430–434, 2001. Available at http://www.cdc.gov/mmwr/preview/mmwrhtml/mm5021a2.htm.

7. Kirchner J: Maternal HIV levels correlate with perinatal transmission. Am Fam Physician 60(9): 3684–3586, 1999.

8. Kuby J: Immunology, 2nd ed. New York, Freeman & Company, 1994.

9. McDonald D, Kuritzkes D: Human immunodeficiency virus type 1 protease inhibitors. Arch Intern Med 157(9):951–959, 1997. Available at http://gateway1.ovid.com/ovidweb.cgi

10. Osmond D: Classification and staging of HIV infection. HIV Insight, 1998. Available at http://hivinsite.ucsf.edu/InSite.jsp?page=kb-01-01#S2X

11. Pilcher C, Eron J, Vemazza P, et al: Sexual transmission during the incubation period of primary HIV infection. JAMA 286 (14):1713–1714, 2001. Available at http://ehostvgw6.epnet.com/ehost

12. Sande M, Volberding P: The Medical Management of AIDS, 3rd ed. Philadelphia, W.B. Saunders, 1992.

3. HEALTH AND PSYCHOSOCIAL ASSESSMENT

Elizabeth Anne Mahoney, RN, MSN, EdD, ACRN

A complete assessment is recommended for comprehensive health care planning for any client and is essential for people who are at risk for or have HIV/AIDS because of the complexity of the condition. The database includes a complete health history (his or her story), physical examination, and laboratory and other diagnostic tests.

1. What are the components of the health history?

The components of the history may vary with agency protocol but usually include the following:

- Biographical data
- Informant
- Reason for contact or seeking care
- Present health or illness
- Past health
- Family history
- Social history
- Daily activities,
- Review of systems

Data should be recorded concisely and systematically, even when the informant may not have followed your sequence, so that all health care providers can readily access the information.

Biographical data include information about who the person is: name, address, telephone number (and if a message can be left), social security number, gender, ethnicity and race, religious preference, health insurance, and health care provider.

The **informant** is the source of the information. Usually the client provides the data. The source and a means for contacting him or her must be listed for future reference and clarification. Other components of the history are discussed in separate questions.

2. What is the difference between the reason for contact or seeking care and present health or illness?

The **reason for contact or seeking care** is a brief statement (no more than a phrase or sentence) in the client's words about the reason for this health encounter. The contact may be wellness-oriented (e.g., an annual examination) or disease-oriented (e.g., a hacking cough that "won't go away"). The reason may or may not be related to HIV/AIDS.

In contrast, **present health or illness** is a statement about positive health, such as "I feel good, no complaints or illnesses." or a detailed symptom analysis of the client's problem:

- Onset
- Duration
- Precipitating or exacerbating factors
- Characteristics of the symptom, such as frequency, amount, duration, and nature (persistent or intermittent; dry, moist, or productive for cough)
- Meaning of the symptom to the client (worrisome, irritating, or does not interfere with work and play)
- Prior occurrence, treatment, and results
- Current treatment and results

This information directs the sequence of the remaining parts of the history, which initially focuses on presenting symptoms and may be abbreviated in emergency situations. Data may indicate that the person has an AIDS-defining condition (e.g., *Mycobacterium avium* complex [MAC]).

Client's words in any record should be brief and placed in quotations marks. These words provide insight into the client's level of understanding and how teaching should be directed.

3. What are the keys parts of the past history?

- Chronic and acute illnesses
- Accidents or injury
- Surgery and hospitalizations
- Childhood diseases
- Immunizations
- Blood transfusions
- Allergies
- Medications (prescription, over-the-counter [OTC], and street drugs)
- Obstetric history for women
- Date of last examination
- Usual frequency of examinations

Dates, where treated, treatment, and sequelae should be provided for all positive responses. These data indicate the presence or absence of practices that promote wellness, complexity of the situation, and consistency of care or "shopping" among providers.

Further, detailed investigation is required for frequent past illnesses (e.g., pneumonia, thrush), sexually transmitted diseases, use of street drugs (especially intravenous drug use), blood transfusion (particularly prior to 1985), and births for women identified with or at risk for HIV/AIDS. If the client has HIV/AIDS, note how it was acquired (if known), when it was diagnosed, past and current treatments, whether the treatment is being followed, treatment progress, and any problems. The frequency of annual health examinations should be verified by asking the date of the last examination.

4. How does the family history contribute to the care of the client?

The family history provides information about the health of family members, the client's risk for familial illnesses, relationships among members, and potential support for the client. A client's risk factors for familial diseases can compound and be compounded by HIV/AIDS. For example, a client with metabolic complications of lipodystrophy syndrome and a family history of diabetes mellitus may be at greater risk for developing diabetes because of glucose intolerance and insulin resistance (see Chapter 14). The client's relationship with family members can help or hinder acceptance of the HIV/AIDS diagnosis. A person who is an integral member of the family is more likely to be supported than one who is already marginalized. Conversely, family members may be at risk if the person with HIV/AIDS lives in the same household or has frequent contact. Disease transmission may occur through shared razors or contact with blood. In addition, if one family member has been abused by another relative, risk for HIV/AIDS should be investigated.

5. Why are social history and daily activities important?

Social history and daily activities include the client's work, school, and recreation activities; relationships with others outside the family; interests; lifestyle; nutritional intake; housing and environment (work and home); finances; and religious, spiritual, and cultural practices. All of these areas provide information about the client as a person, risks for disease, potential sources of support, and factors that influence a treatment regimen positively or negatively. For example, is the client returning to a setting that fostered acquisition of HIV/AIDS?

6. Why is the review of systems important?

The review of systems (ROS) is the last component of the health history. Because of the similarity in areas reviewed, many confuse the ROS with the physical examination (PE). The subjective data of the ROS provide the opportunity to review the past and present state of all body systems, to ensure that all relevant data are collected, and to determine wellness-promotive practices.[2] The presence or absence of each item in the ROS must be recorded, so that readers do not have to question whether the information was denied or not reviewed.

7. What are the similarities and differences between the ROS and the PE?

The main similarity between the ROS and the PE is the collection of data about all body systems. The major difference is the technique for data collection. The ROS is based on what is said (**subjective data**), whereas PE data are collected by inspection, palpation, percussion, and/or auscultation (**objective data**). The history data provide the signposts for the PE, pointing to particular areas that require attention. Together they direct the use of laboratory and other diagnostic tests to determine the nature of the client's problem(s) and ultimately the treatment regimen.

8. What are key subjective and objective data to collect for clients with or at risk for HIV/AIDS?[3,6,8]

A complete history and PE should be conducted for all clients. Components are clearly presented in any health or physical assessment textbook. The information here focuses on data of particular relevance for people with HIV/AIDS. ROS and PE data are provided for each area/system as subjective (S) or objective (O), respectively.

The first ROS (S) information collected relates to the person's **general health status**: current height and weight (along with recent planned or unplanned changes), fatigue, malaise or weakness, fever, chills, sweats (especially night sweats, which suggest the potential for *Mycobacterium tuberculosis)*. Weight change (gain or loss), fatigue, and fever are common complaints and may indicate HIV/AIDS-related conditions, such as lymphomas or wasting.

PE (O) data relate to age, gender, appearance, behavior and affect, general body state, posture, gait, actual height and weight, and vital signs. Results can support (weight loss) or negate (afebrile) the client's description.

Each system is reviewed with the client in detail. Common elements for all S data include pain or discomfort, family history, past history of illness or injuries to the body area, change or loss of function, assistive devices, coping measures, and wellness-promotive behaviors. Common assessments for O data relate to symmetry, presence of masses or lesions and their descriptions, swelling, color, missing or altered body part or function, adaptive devices and their use/results, altered sounds, and altered odors.

9. Identify the appropriate data related to skin, hair, and nails.

S: changes in pigmentation, lesions, pruritus; hair loss or change in texture; nails and parenchyma.

O: dryness, dermatitis, red/black lesions that do not blanch on pressure (Kaposi's sarcoma), fungal or viral infections or lesions.

10. What are the appropriate data for the head, nose, mouth, throat, sinuses, and neck?

S: headaches; mouth, gum, and pharyngeal discomfort or sores; burning sensation when drinking fruit juices; lymph node swelling; kind and frequency of dental care.

O: white plaques in the oropharynx that become red or bleed when scraped, peridontal disease, lymphadenopathy.

11. Summarize the appropriate data for the eyes and ears.

Eyes

S: change in visual acuity or fields, "floaters," frequency and date of last eye examination.

O: decreased visual acuity on Snellen chart, unilateral visual field loss, retinal lesions.

Ears

S: ear pain, discharge, hearing change or loss.

O: results of whisper, Weber, and Rinne tests; otoscopic visualization.

12. What are the appropriate data for the thorax and lungs?

S: cough (productive/nonproductive), sputum and its characteristics, dyspnea at rest and on exertion, history of or exposure to tuberculosis, pneumonia, last chest x-ray and results.

O: respiratory rate and characteristics, cough, sputum, adventitious breath sounds.

13. Describe the appropriate data related to the cardiovascular and peripheral vascular systems.

S: past/family history of disease, diet, chest pain, shortness of breath, numbness, tingling, burning, coldness in extremities.

O: heart rate, rhythm, and sounds; temperature; color and distribution of hair on extremities; lesions; capillary refill; upper and lower extremity pulses.

14. Describe the appropriate data related to the abdomen and gastrointestinal system.

S: nausea, vomiting, diarrhea, constipation; change in or loss of appetite; pain and difficulty with swallowing; feeling of food "stuck in" chest; rectal bleeding; last colonoscopy.

O: hyper- or hypoactive bowel sounds, dullness versus tympany; pain on palpation; hepatosplenomegaly; inguinal lymphadenopathy.

15. What data should be included in relation to the breasts (female and male)?

S: pain or discomfort, masses; drainage from nipples; breast self-examination (time of month, frequency, method, results); last mammography, usual frequency, and results.

O: symmetry, masses, dimpling, nipple discharge, lymphadenopathy.

16. What data are important in relation to the genitourinary system and sexual history?

S: dysuria, frequency, burning, itching, nocturia, change in urine characteristics; genital lesions, discharge, diseases (and treatment).

For men: testicular self-examination (frequency, time, method).

For women: menstrual and obstetric history, menorrhagia, metrorrhagia, gynecologic examination (frequency, results of Papanicolaou [Pap] smear).

For both genders: anal sex, anorectal examination (frequency and results).

S: current and past sexual practices (active or inactive; monogamous or multiple partners; homo-, hetero-, or bisexual relations of self or partner[s]; oral, genital, and anal sex; protected sex with condoms or other means; history and treatment of sexually transmitted diseases or HIV/AIDS for self, present partner, and other partners).

O: inspect and palpate external genitalia for masses and lesions; note and culture drainage; anorectal examination; palpate for hernia in men; gynecologic examination with Pap smear in women.

17. Summarize the appropriate data related to the musculoskeletal system.

S: pain or discomfort, swelling in joints and muscles; bone pain or deformity; asymmetry; decreased muscle strength or range of joint motion.

O: asymmetry (size, contour, color, characteristics), decreased range of motion; swelling or masses in muscles or joints; decreased muscle strength.

18. Describe the appropriate data related to the neurologic system.

S: mental status (changes in memory, attention, level of consciousness); sensory status (peripheral neuropathies, pain); motor status (impaired walking, tremors, palsy, weakness, fatigue); cerebellar status (dizziness, vertigo); cranial nerves (visual/sensory deficits).

O: Mental status (deficits in memory, attention, level of consciousness); sensory deficits; motor status (impaired walking or activities of daily living, hemiparesis, tremors, palsy, weakness, fatigue); cerebellar status (imbalance); cranial nerves (visual/sensory deficits, altered speech); reflexes (diminished or no change).

19. What data are important in relation to the hematologic system?

S: easy bruising, bleeding, swelling of lymph nodes.

O: bruising, lymphadenopathy.

20. What data are important in relation to the endocrine system:
   S: personal or family history of diabetes or thyroid disease; excessive thirst or hunger; void-
ing; altered hair distribution.
   O: soft skin, abnormal hair distribution.

**21. Summarize the subjective and objective data that may indicate major opportunistic in-
fections and malignancies associated with HIV/AIDS.**

BODY AREA/ SYSTEM	SUBJECTIVE DATA	OBJECTIVE DATA	POTENTAL DISORDER
General health status	Fever > 30 days Fatigue Lethargy Weakness Weight loss	Fever Weight loss > 10% Diarrhea	HIV wasting*
Other systems	Decreased activity Anorexia, nausea, vomiting, diarrhea	Decreased muscle mass/ atrophy	
General health status	Fever > 2 wk Chills Night sweats Weight loss No pain	Enlarged lymph nodes Varied symptoms (depending on areas affected CD4 < 200/mm³ X-ray/biopsy results	Non-Hodgkin's lymphoma*
General health status	Fever Weight loss Night sweats	Fever Mouth ulcers Hepatomegaly Splenomegaly	Histoplasmosis*
Other systems	Mouth sores Shortness of breath Exposure to fungal con- tamination of soil, soil, bird or bat droppings	Gastrointestinal ulcers Diffuse infiltrate on x-ray CD4 < 50/mm³ Anemia Leukopenia Positive blood/bone marrow cultures	
General health status	Fever, especially of un- known origin Fatigue Malaise Night sweats Weight loss	Weight loss Hepatomegaly Splenomegaly Lymphadenopathy Low CD4 count Anemia	*Mycobacterium avium* complex, *M. avium-intra- cellulare* complex*
Other systems	Abdominal pain Anorexia Diarrhea	Elevated alkaline phosphatase Blood and sputum cultures positive for organism	
Skin	"Bruises," lumps on face, in mouth, on chest and genitals No pain, itching	Blue-red lesions (progress from macules/papules to to patches/plaques to nodules to vascular tumor) No blanching when pressed Eventually spread to organs, producing related symptoms	Kaposi's sarcoma*
Eyes	Asymptomatic or "floaters" Decreased visual acuity Unilateral visual field loss, progressing to bilateral field loss and blindness	Decreased visual acuity Unilateral visual field loss Retinal lesions CD4 count < 50/mm³	Cytomegalovirus*

Table continued on following page

BODY AREA/ SYSTEM	SUBJECTIVE DATA	OBJECTIVE DATA	POTENTIAL DISORDER
Mouth and throat	Painless white patches in mouth, throat, tongue "Burning" when acids (e.g., juices) are swallowed Soreness and bleeding of mouth and tongue if patches removed	White, cheese-like plaques on buccal and pharyngeal mucosa and tongue Bleeding when plaque scraped Also redness in mouth, pharynx, tongue	Candidiasis (thrush)
Respiratory	Increased dyspnea on exertion Nonproductive cough	Increased respirations Nonspecific adventitious breath sounds Bilateral interstitial infiltrate CD4 < 200 mm^3	*Pneumocystis carinii pneumonia**
Respiratory	Dyspnea Productive cough Blood-tinged sputum	Productive cough Blood-tinged sputum	*Mycobacterium tuberculosis**
Other systems	Fever, chills Malaise Night sweats Weight loss	Fever, chills Weight loss Sputum culture positive for acid-fast bacillus	
GI tract Esophagus	Pain and difficulty with swallowing (dysphagia) Feeling of food stuck in chest	Possibly thrush CD4 < 200 mm^3	Candidiasis (esophagus),* CMV,* or herpes zoster
Female genitalia/ sexual health	Multiple sex partners Unprotected intercourse Human papillomavirus Early: asymptomatic Bleeding between menses and/or after coitus Blood-tinged vaginal discharge with foul odor	Squamous cell abnormalities on biopsy	Cervical intraepithelial neoplasia or cervical cancer (stage III)*
Female genitalia/ sexual health	Pruritus Increased bleeding during and between menses White or yellow cheese-like discharge	Redness and swelling of external genitalia White or yellow cheese-like discharge	Vaginal candidiasis
Neurologic	Numbness, tingling, burning, prickling sensation of skin/feet in prior herpes zoster site (e.g., balls of feet); may progress upward Impaired walking due to discomfort	Impaired walking	Peripheral neuropathy Herpes zoster neuralgia
Neurologic	Decreased concentration Forgetfulness	Decreased mental acuity, concentration, attention, new learning Impaired motor function/ activities of daily living Absence of CNS opportunistic infections	Encephalopathy AIDS dementia complex*

Table continued on following page

BODY AREA/ SYSTEM	SUBJECTIVE DATA	OBJECTIVE DATA	POTENTIAL DISORDER
Neurologic	Headaches Vertigo Seizures Mental, sensory, motor, visual deficits	Mental, sensory, motor, visual deficits CD4 < 90/mm^3 CT scan abnormalities Brain biopsy data Positive JCV[5]	Progressive multifocal leukoencepha-lopathy*
Neurologic	Initially asymptomatic Headache Weakness, fatigue Dizziness Altered level of conscious-ness Tremors, CNS palsy	Altered level of consciousness Tremors, CNS palsy Weakness Hemiparesis Lymphadenopathy Low-grade fever Abnormal speech	Toxoplasmosis*
Other systerms	Low-grade fever Malaise	CD4 < 100/mm^3	

CMV = cytomegalovrius, GI = gastrointestinal, CNS = central nervous system, JCV = JC virus.
* AIDS-defining conditions.[1]

22. What are the more common laboratory and diagnostic tests associated with defining and treating HIV/AIDS?

The usual tests to confirm, treat, and monitor HIV/AIDS include complete blood count (CBC) and chemistries, CD4 cell counts, viral load assays, and genotype or phenotype resistance tests. Common tests for related disorders or sequelae include lipid profiles; testosterone levels for men; serologic testing for syphilis, *Toxoplasma gondii*, cytomegalovirus, and anti-varicella IgG (chicken pox); screening for tuberculosis and hepatitis A, B and C; chest x-ray; and CT scan.[7]

23. Which patients should be questioned about sexual health? Are they comfortable or uncomfortable in talking about such personal matters?

HIV and sexually transmitted diseases do not discriminate by age, gender, ethnic or religious background, education, or financial status. Therefore, all persons who are presently or potentially sexually active or who use drugs should be questioned about sexual health. The chapters on epidemiology and vulnerable populations illustrate the scope of HIV/AIDS.

The sexual history comes later in the data collection and affords the interviewer the opportunity to promote a nonjudgmental, caring, helpful environment in which the client can honestly respond to personal questions without fear of censure.[1] Nurses must examine their own attitudes toward people who have different lifestyles and encourage open dialogue that fosters a positive nurse–patient relationship and optimal client care.

Some clients are quite comfortable with discussing their personal experiences, and the nurse may be the one who is uncomfortable with talking about sexual activities or drug behaviors. Again, nurses must become aware of and deal with their biases so that they do not become barriers to effective care. Nurses cannot make clients disclose information that they wish to withhold. Nurses who are uncomfortable talking with clients about their personal behaviors can role-play the interview to minimize negative responses before collecting data from a client.

A complete database (history, physical examination, and laboratory and other diagnostic data) gives health care providers the information that they need to provide holistic health care and promote the client's adherence to interventions that minimize the effects of HIV/AIDS. Components of the database are discussed in greater detail in subsequent chapters.

BIBLIOGRAPHY

1. Barrett JG, Gallant JC: 2001–2003 Medical Management of HIV Infection. Baltimore, Johns Hopkins University Press, 2001.
2. Capili B, Anastasi, JK: Assess for HIV, too. RN 61(4), 28-32, 1998. Available at http://gateway2.ovid.com/ovidweb.cgi
3. Jarvis C: Physical Examination and Health Assessment, 3rd ed. Philadelphia, W.B. Saunders, 2000.
4. Kirton CA, Talotta D, Zwolski K: Handbook of HIV/AIDS Nursing. St. Louis, Mosby, 2001.
5. Ropka ME, Williams AB: HIV Nursing and Symptom Management. Boston, Jones & Bartlett, 1998.
6. The seropositive patient—The initial encounter: The initial history and physical exam. Medscape Today, 2002. Available at http://www.medscape.com/viewarticle/421503_4.
7. The seropositive patient—The initial encounter: Laboratory studies. Medscape Today, 2002. Available at http://www.medscape.com/viewarticle/421503_5.
8. Ungvarski PJ, Flaskerud JH: HIV/AIDS: A Guide to Primary Care Management, 4th ed. Philadelphia, W.B. Saunders, 1999.

4. ADHERENCE TO TREATMENT PLAN

Judy K. Shaw, MS, ACRN, ANP-C

Adherence, especially in relationship to medications, has been a key emphasis in HIV/AIDS for several years. The reason is simple: medications, no matter how efficacious or therapeutic, simply do not work if they are not taken properly. The nurse plays an essential role in promoting patient adherence by providing education, initiating behavior change, advocating for patient rights, and providing social support.

1. Describe adherence. Why is it important?

Adherence encompasses all activities necessary to achieve the most positive outcome possible for each patient. Medication adherence is a major part of the overall picture. What we know now about antiretroviral medications is quite simple: if they are not taken properly, they will not work. Proper and consistent dosing is necessary to maintain therapeutic levels and to achieve and maintain optimal viral suppression. For some antiretroviral medications, dietary restrictions must be followed to ensure that serum levels of the medication remain at the proper level and to decrease the likelihood of adverse side effects.

In addition to taking medications properly, adherence requires keeping clinic appointments, undergoing required tests, and following a personalized plan of care. For some patients, adherence might include keeping appointments with a mental health counselor and taking the medications that he or she prescribes. For others, maintaining sobriety is part of adherence. Regular eye exams and up-to-date immunizations are all part of the health plan and require adherence.

Positive patient outcomes should be a priority for health care providers. However, in the case of HIV/AIDS, poor adherence with medication protocol can result in something more serious than one patient's failure to do well. Studies have shown that poor antiretroviral adherence leads to viral resistance.[1-3] A growing concern in the scientific community is that a resistant strain of HIV/AIDS could develop, as has occurred with other diseases.

2. How can providers know that someone is resistant to antiretroviral medications?

Cases have been reported of patients newly diagnosed with HIV who already have resistant mutations when they are tested because the person by whom they were infected had viral mutations as a result of poor response to therapy and viral breakthrough or nonadherence. Genotypic and phenotypic assays are becoming more widely used to measure resistance to antiretroviral agents. Genotypic resistance assays involve DNA sequencing and report mutations for each gene. Phenotypic assays report susceptibility to medications. Some data suggest which medications are less likely to work in the presence of certain mutations; thus, these tests can help to guide the provider's choices in selecting initial therapy or changes in therapy. Because limited data are available about the efficacy of prescribing therapy based solely on genotypic or phenotypic results, clinical presentation and past medication history must be carefully considered in recommending any antiretroviral therapy.

3. What is the difference between adherence and compliance?

Compliance means simply to follow instructions. "The doctor says that I have to take this pill three times a day." The patient may or may not know the purpose of the pill or on what basis the decision was made. Compliance reflects a paternalistic paradigm in which patients do what they are told because someone who knows better has given them instructions to do so.

Adherence is a more holistic, patient-centered approach to therapy. Possible options are discussed with the patient, along with the pros and cons of each, and a mutually agreed upon plan is developed. Education is a key component of a good adherence program and allows patients to make informed decisions based on accurate and up-to-date information.

Plans should be individualized to specific patient needs and lifestyles. For example, someone who works the second shift and does not go to bed until early morning on work days should not be expected to get up to take the first dose of medication at 6 AM. A plan that is mismatched to the patient will result in missed medication doses, discouragement on the part of the patient, and overall poor outcome.

4. How strictly should adherence be defined?

Everyone knows from personal experience that there are times when a patient simply does not take medication—for whatever reason. The question, then, is how many doses can be missed before the likelihood of viral breakthrough increases? Does it really matter if a patient does not take the medication every Friday night because he is going out with friends and knows that he should not mix it with alcohol? What about the person who forgets to renew the prescription at the pharmacy and does not take any medication for four days?

Recently, researchers investigating the effect of missed doses of medication on viral suppression found a statistically significant improvement in viral suppression as the degree of adherence increased.[1] The percentage of participants with an undetectable viral load dropped by 20% when adherence decreased from 95–100% to 95–90%. Consider a person who takes pills 3 times/day. If he or she misses seven doses of medication in one month, the likelihood of having an undetectable viral load decreases from 100% to 80%. Even more surprisingly, the number of participants with an undetectable viral load dropped to almost half when adherence decreased from 95-100% to 80-90%. The results of this study emphasize the magnitude of the problem associated with nonadherence—especially since overall estimates suggest that between 30% and 90% of people with any chronic illness do not adhere to their medication regimen.

5. What makes adherence so difficult?

Adherence to any plan involves making a decision and commitment to change behavior patterns. The majority of people, in general, find it difficult to do the same thing at the same time every day with little fluctuation. In addition, many factors specific to HIV/AIDS make adherence to medications and the treatment plan difficult.

First, although anyone can become infected with HIV/AIDS, most persons infected worldwide belong to minority groups who are often financially and socially deprived. Many have limited resources and social support systems. Something as "simple" as finding transportation to a clinic can be very difficult, depending on the patient's situation. During times when close monitoring or additional tests are needed, it can be especially difficult juggling transportation and caretaking needs. For many women, taking care of themselves is not their highest priority; they may have additional caretaking responsibilities for children, partners, or other family members who are also infected. Lack of education, cultural differences, homelessness, poor coping skills, and financial need make access to adequate health care difficult.

Medication adherence is complicated because multiple dosing and dietary restrictions are required. Patients taking a typical combination therapy and prophylaxis for *Pneumocystis carinii* pneumonia and *Mycobacterium avium* complex may take more than 30 pills/day or 200 pills/week. Some medications must be taken with food and others on an empty stomach. Some require the patient to consume 8 glasses/day of water. Some can be taken once daily, others twice daily, and still others 3 times/day. Azidothymidine (AZT), the first widely used antiretroviral medication, was originally taken 5 times/day. Some patients plan much of the day around taking medications properly. Others need to make lifestyle changes to allow them to be adherent.

6. How have pharmaceutical companies responded to problems with adherence?

Within the past few years, pharmaceutical companies have realized how importance adherence is to patient outcomes. In response, efforts have been made to simplify dosing schedules and decrease pill burden. Currently two pills on the market are combinations of two or three medications in one tablet to lower pill burden: Combivir (epivir and AZT) and Trizivir (epivir, AZT, and abacavir). Several medications can now safely be taken fewer times per day by increasing the dosage or adding another medication that has a synergistic effect (i.e., ritonavir). Currently, certain regimens consist of as few as 5 pills/day with a twice-daily dosing schedule and many fewer dietary restrictions.

7. How does use of street drugs complicate adherence?

Although antiretroviral therapy is not contraindicated in persons who are actively using street drugs, users' lifestyles are more chaotic and tend to result in a higher incidence of nonadherence. From a public health viewpoint, promoting adherence in this group is especially important because the use of street drugs and alcohol can lead to increased sexual activity with multiple partners and a greater chance of viral transmission and infection with HIV.

8. What role do side effects play in adherence?

For many patients, unwanted side effects are the greatest barrier to medication adherence. Diarrhea, nausea, and vomiting are not uncommon, especially for the first few weeks after initiating a new therapy. Patients also may have many other side effects, including vivid dreams or nightmares, rash, elevation in liver enzymes, anemia, or neutropenia. In some cases, side effects may be so severe that therapy must be changed or stopped altogether.

9. What are the most common reasons that patients cite for nonadherence?[4]

- Too many pills to manage
- Falling asleep before night doses
- Being away from home longer than expected without medications
- Use of alcohol and/or drugs
- Medications lost or stolen
- No insurance
- Forgetting to call for refills
- Unexpected change in routine
- Mental illness, including depression and conscious choice not to take medications
- Need for a break (medication holiday) for a few days/weeks
- Simple forgetfulness

10. Do we know why some people are adherent with their care plan and others are not?

It is impossible to say what makes a person follow a plan to treat disease and promote wellness. Some people are simply not willing to make lifestyle changes. Others are willing to compromise to a point but will not violate preset limits. People may be in denial or feel as though they want to live their life to the fullest and let fate decide their destiny. Many want to do what is right, but circumstances prevent them from doing so. Some people still do not believe that AIDS is caused by HIV. On the other hand, some persons vow adherence and want to live as long and as well as possible at any cost.

In one recent study,[5] sociodemographic and psychological factors were examined to see whether any trends could be identified. The greatest number of adherent participants were in their 30s, did not have a history of depression or intravenous drug use, felt that they had a good social support system, and had CD4 cells in the 200–499 range when they began antiretroviral therapy.

11. What are the possible effects of nonadherence on personal and public health?

Nonadherence has several possible negative outcomes. Primarily it leads to decreases in CD4 count, which indicate a greater degree of immunosuppression and an increase in viral load. Low CD4 counts have been correlated with a greater likelihood of developing an opportunistic or other acute infection, an increase in hospital admissions, and more rapid progression to AIDS and death. A viral load above the level of detection (currently < 50 copies) increases the risk of HIV transmission proportionately to the copies of virus detected. Patients with lower CD4 counts and higher viral loads have reported a decreased perception of quality of life.

In addition to individual negative patient outcomes, nonadherence can lead to development of resistant strains of HIV, as has already happened with tuberculosis (TB) and vancomycin-resistant enterococcus (VRE). The fact that resistant mutations are present in newly diagnosed cases of HIV emphasizes the importance of adherence.

12. What can be done to make adherence easier?

Although there are no easy answers, a number of interventions have been shown to help and correlate well with the reasons for nonadherence cited by patients.[6] In each case, nurses can be instrumental in advocating for patients and initiating change.

1. The **basic essentials for survival, such as food, clothing, and shelter,** must be provided before patients can make lifestyle changes. This point may seem simplistic, but a homeless person who must rely on food pantries or soup kitchens for meals has difficulty with managing a therapy regimen requiring multiple dosing and dietary restrictions. Like addicts who are totally consumed by the desire to "get their fix," homeless people must forage for food, clothing, and a safe place to sleep. Even if someone is not homeless, a chaotic lifestyle (e.g., multiple people living in one space, abuse of alcohol and/or drugs) contributes to the inability to maintain a medication regimen. If possible, the patient should be helped to secure adequate, safe housing, a steady source of food, and social support before beginning therapy. This is not possible in all cases, especially if the patient is very sick or at risk for developing opportunistic infections. Still, a stable lifestyle has been shown to improve the likelihood of adherence.

2. **Education** is also a key component. Patients cannot be expected to endorse a plan until they are able to understand why it is important and what choices are available. Even a basic understanding of the disease process can have a positive impact on adherence and prevention strategies. New HIV/AIDS-related material or a review of material already covered during previous visits should be presented by the nurse at each visit. Time should be allowed for questions and answer. Open, honest discussions contribute to the nurse-patient relationship and overall feeling of security and can be a source of personal support for patients.

3. **Referrals to community-based organizations or faith communities that specialize in HIV/AIDS** are important. These organizations often provide services such as support groups, aggregate dining, social functions, activist meetings, and assistance with legal issues. Involvement provides patients with the opportunity to meet people who are facing similar problems and life situations and to develop a network of social support in the community.

4. **Flexibility** is important for patients who have difficulty with fitting into a set clinic schedule. Flexible scheduling, including walk-in, evening, and weekend clinic hours, allows options that fit into most schedules. The availability of a nurse by phone to answer questions and to triage patient needs contributes to continuity of care and decreases visits to emergency departments.

5. **Numerous assistive devices** are available to aid in medication adherence, including pill boxes, devices set to alarm at dosing times, charts, and phone reminder services. Before any plan is developed, a thorough investigation should be made into the patient's lifestyle to determine individual needs. Home visits by the nurse can be especially helpful in obtaining an overall view that includes cultural, social, and economic needs. General recommendations are available, but a specialized plan should be developed for each patient to ensure that specific needs are addressed.

13. Does an increase in viral load always mean that the patient is not adherent?

No. A rise in viral load can occur for several different reasons, but nonadherence should always be the first consideration. Although it is important to be accepting and trust the patient, nonadherence is one area in which people may be hesitant to be honest. Two main reasons are to avoid being "scolded" and to avoid the provider's "anger" at the patient's failure to follow through. Other patients obviously recognize the effort put forth by providers and nurses and do not want to "disappoint" them. Frequent follow-up in person or by phone provides support and assurance to patients who struggle with adherence.

Another reason for a rise in viral load is viral breakthrough, which occurs when the virus mutates to the point that the antiretroviral medications are no longer effective. When resistance occurs, there is usually a gradual upward trend in viral load rather than a sharp, sudden rise. Regular monitoring allows early detection of changes in viral load.

Occasionally, patients have an isolated rise in the number of copies of virus on a viral load test. The cause for these "blips," as they are called in the literature, may not always be identified, but usually they are attributed to intermittent periods of nonadherence, testing variance, or lab error. A repeat of the viral load in 2–3 weeks usually helps to determine whether the increase is a sign of developing resistance or attributable to one of the causes listed above.

14. What is the nurse's role in promoting adherence?

The nurse is an essential part of the adherence team. Using nursing theories that incorporate a holistic approach, the nurse is able to assess the physiologic and psychosocial needs of the patient, assist in developing and implementing a care plan, and actively evaluate outcomes. The nurse works collaboratively with other disciplines to coordinate services for the patient. In many cases, the nurse has the greatest number and most frequent interactions with the patient. Frequent follow-up and support provided by the health team have been shown to promote adherence and to have a significant impact on the overall outcome of the patient.[6]

BIBLIOGRAPHY

1. Eldred L, Wu A, Chaisson R, Moore R: Adherence to antiretroviral and pneumocystis prophylaxis in HIV disease. J Acq Immune Defic Hum Retrovirol 18:117–125, 1998.
2. Gordeillo V, del Amo J, Soriano V, Gonzalez-Lahoz J: Sociodemographic and psychological variables influencing adherence to antiretroviral therapy. AIDS 13: 1763–1769, 1999.
3. Knobel H, Carmona A, Grau S, et al: Adherence and effectiveness of highly active antiretroviral therapy. Arch Intern Med 158:1953, 1998.
4. Low-Beer S, Yip B, O'Shaughnessy M, et al: Adherence to triple therapy and the viral load response. J Acq Immune Defici Syndr 23(4):360, 2000.
5. Paterson D, Swindells S, Mohr J, et al: Adherence to protease inhibitor therapy and outcomes in patients with HIV infection. Ann Intern Med133:21–30, 2000.
6. Reiter G, Stewart K, Wojtusik L, et al: Elements of success in HIV clinical care: Multiple interventions that promote adherence. Int AIDS Soc 8(5):21–30, 2000.

5. NURSING CARE OF PATIENTS WITH HIV/AIDS

Inge B. Corless, RN, PhD, FAAN, and Patrice K. Nicholas, RN, DNSc, ANP, MPH

In the beginning of the HIV/AIDS pandemic, when epidemiologists were tracking the first few cases identified as a suspicious new disease and physicians were attempting to treat a disease for which they had no known cure, nurses were present to provide care. Not all nurses, of course— some, like other providers, were reluctant or refused to give care. We have come a long way since those early days. Options for treatment are now available and have modified the content of nursing care. But the importance of nursing care remains unchanged, for it is the nurse who works with the patient to ensure that the gains of science are translated into the benefits of care.

1. Who is the patient?

The patient is a person who is infected or has the potential to be infected with the human immunodeficiency virus (HIV) and the partner and family of the infected person. It may seem obvious that people already infected are seen as patients and that for nurses the family is also a focus of interest. For nurses, however, potentially infected people are also "patients" or, better yet, "clients" because they will be seen for counseling and testing. Furthermore, given that all people have the potential for infection, the nurse who is active in health promotion works to educate people about ways to prevent infection with HIV. With HIV disease, the nurse's role involves education for prevention of HIV transmission, care of the infected person, and education and support of partners and family. How the patient is defined depends on the nurse's role at a specific time.

2. What are the goals of nursing care for the HIV-positive person?

The goals of nursing care are aimed at assessment, treatment, and education of people at risk and people already infected with HIV. Subjective data include a thorough review of risk factors, history, and review of systems. The physical examination should focus carefully on the mouth, eyes, skin, lungs, heart, lymph nodes, abdomen, central and peripheral nervous system, genitalia, and rectum. An in-depth laboratory and diagnostic evaluation is included in the plan of care. The thorough assessment leads to diagnosis and treatment of HIV-related conditions and prevention of opportunistic infections. Education about the chronic nature of HIV disease and social and psychological aspects of care should include the HIV-positive person and the family/significant others. Medication issues include the risks and benefits of delayed initiation of therapy and early therapy in the HIV-positive person. Discussion of adherence to medication and management of side effects of medications are essential in the care of the HIV-positive person. Nutrition issues, a healthy lifestyle, and prevention of transmission of HIV are additional important issues in the nursing care of the HIV-positive person.

In addition, specific goals of HIV therapy and tools to achieve these goals have been identified in the most recent *Guidelines for the Use of Antiretroviral Agents in HIV-infected Adults and Adolescents*. These guidelines indicate the following specific goals of antiretroviral therapy:

- Maximal and durable suppression of viral load
- Restoration and/or preservation of immunologic function
- Improvement of quality of life
- Reduction of HIV-related morbidity and mortality

Based on these guidelines, the tools to achieve the goals of therapy are as follows:

- Maximizing adherence to the antiretroviral regimen
- Rational sequencing of drugs
- Preservation of future treatment options
- Resistance testing in selected clinical settings.

3. How can the nurse incorporate the nursing process into the plan of care?

The nursing process includes assessment, diagnosis, planning, implementation/intervention, and evaluation. These elements of the nursing process are critical aspects of the process for care of the person with HIV.

Assessment takes place during the nurse's first encounter with the client and continues throughout the nurse/client relationship. Assessment of the person with HIV involves the collection of relevant data from the client, family/significant other, medical records, and diagnostic test results. Assessment may include data from the review of systems, family dynamics, cultural issues, and community resources. Both subjective and objective data are important in the assessment process. Subjective data come directly from the client (e.g., health history); objective data include physical examination findings and laboratory results.

Diagnosis is applicable to the patient with HIV both for formulating nursing diagnoses and for considering the medical diagnoses that affect persons with HIV. Nursing diagnoses are often related to symptom management, including diagnoses related to altered nutrition, pain, potential for infection, body image disturbance, diarrhea, and ineffective coping. The role of the nurse also includes addressing the patient's medical diagnoses and planning nursing care based on these.

Planning requires that the nurse develop a plan based on the diagnoses that will help the person with HIV to achieve optimal functioning. The plan of care must be tailored to the client and realistic for the specific client's needs. The nurse must recognize the needs of the HIV client and family, including their strengths and weaknesses. Setting goals is a mutual process involving both nurse and client and often includes family members or significant others. Determining priorities of care is an important part of this process, allowing the HIV infected person to retain as much control as possible of his or her health.

Intervention and implementation follow the phase of setting goals and selecting plans, including decisions about when or whether to start medications.

Evaluation occurs throughout the intervention phase and is linked to the outcome criteria established for patient goals. For example, if the intervention for a person with HIV includes initiating antiretroviral therapy, evaluation should include monitoring of adherence, follow-up on markers of therapy (viral load and other diagnostic studies), and quality-of-life issues.

4. How can the nurse establish a therapeutic alliance with the patient?

The therapeutic alliance is an important element in developing a relationship with the person living with HIV. Beginning with the initial encounter, the nurse must establish a climate of trust to promote the interaction necessary for developing a therapeutic relationship focused on the client's needs. Creating a climate of trust from the initial encounter requires that the client be empowered as an active participant in the therapeutic alliance. In a successful therapeutic alliance, addressing the client's specific needs, jointly developing a plan of care, and contracting for client goals can be discussed. For example, if the HIV-positive client is going to start antiretroviral therapy, a verbal or written contract can be developed between the nurse and client.

5. What is the role of the nurse during the initial visit of the HIV-positive person?

During the initial visit, the health care provider is likely to order a repeat HIV diagnostic test, usually an enzyme-linked immunosorbent assay (ELISA) screening confirmed by a Western blot assay if the repeat ELISA is positive. A number of stories are told about patients being treated for HIV disease on the basis of a patient report, only to find on a repeat test that the person is negative. This problem has less to do with the accuracy of the test than with the integrity of the patient or, on rare occasions, the accuracy of the laboratory. At any rate, good practice requires verification of the diagnosis. The role of the nurse is to educate the patient about the need for such verification and what information about health status various tests provide. For this reason the practitioner may decide to do a viral load test, either polymerase chain reaction (PCR) or branched DNA (bDNA), rather than a repeat antibody test. The viral load indicates the current level of virus replication in the plasma. In most instances, both antibody and viral load tests are required.

In addition to educating the patient about HIV testing, the nurse must assess the patient's social history, including sexual activities, needle exposure, family history, and use of mood-affecting drugs. The health care provider should also ascertain the patient's history of immunizations, sexually transmitted diseases, medical diagnosis, medications, occupations, and women's diseases, as appropriate. Assessment for hepatitis A, B, and C, as well as tuberculosis, is an important part of the health history. Investigating access to insurance is essential as part of the initial visit, so that the patient has the financial support necessary for treatment and for daily living, if additional support is needed for more than illness-related expenses. The nurse can be very helpful in advocating for the patient for needed financial resources.

6. What are the components of holistic care for the person living with HIV/AIDS?

Holistic care for the person with HIV should always focus on health promotion and maintenance, addressing culture and ethnicity, including alternative and complementary therapies. Holistic care includes promoting a healthy lifestyle and behaviors that prolong the asymptomatic stage of HIV infection and limit the occurrence of opportunistic infections. Holistic care also includes prophylaxis and treatment of opportunistic infections, rehabilitation, and palliative care across the spectrum of HIV disease.

7. What question do you need answered before the patient leaves?

The vital question to be discussed is with whom the patient plans to share the information about his or her HIV status. It is important to identify the patient's source of support, who may or may not be the partner or spouse. Some people with HIV may incur physical harm if the partner or spouse is informed. Then the issue is to ascertain alternative sources of support. Assessing the patient's ability to cope with a new HIV diagnosis during the visit is essential to the patient's future well-being, as is securing appropriate mental health and social support referrals. The patient's plan for self-care at this time is crucial information. Furthermore, written material, as appropriate, provides reinforcement of patient education. Lastly, having the patient call in to report how things are going (or having the nurse call at an appropriate time) is helpful for the newly diagnosed client. Care must be taken, however, so that the phone call does not provoke unwanted inquiries by significant and insignificant others.

8. What do patients need to know to live with HIV/AIDS?

Patients need to know that HIV is a chronic disease that progresses from initial exposure to asymptomatic HIV infection, symptomatic HIV infection, and AIDS. Medication therapy can slow the progression of HIV and limit the opportunistic infections that arise as the immune system becomes depleted. HIV disease has a variable course in different people. Factors related to HIV transmission and disease progression are important for patients to learn, primarily to prevent transmission of disease to other persons. Living with HIV requires that the HIV-positive person focus on a health-promoting diet, regular exercise, and avoidance of stress and substance use. The issues of transmission of HIV during childbearing also must be discussed, if appropriate.

9. What resources may the nurse help the patient access?

In addition to financial resources for medications, patients with HIV/AIDS may not have stable housing situations. Securing stable housing is essential for most people, especially when there is the need to take medications on a regular basis. In addition, providing the name, address, and phone number of community-based organizations helps the patient obtain a range of support, including the companionship of others with the same diagnosis. Some community organizations provide special services, such as acupuncture and massage. Each community differs in the range of services that are available. The nurse should investigate the range of available services to provide the necessary support to the HIV-infected client.

10. How does prevention apply when the client is already infected?

Although the client is infected with HIV, prevention is still a significant part of health teaching. First, as part of the initial visit, it is important to educate the patient about how not to transmit

HIV infection to sexual or needle-sharing partners. A feeling in some communities is that everyone should look out for him- or herself. This individualistic perspective is diametrically opposed to the communitarian approach that each person has responsibility for others. In a communitarian society, what we do has an impact, for better or worse, on those around us. A community-minded person wants the impact to be for the better, realizing his or her responsibility even to the unknown other. From this perspective, the HIV-infected person needs to take precautions, either by abstinence or by the use of condoms and/or clean works (intravenous injection equipment), to avoid transmission of HIV infection. Since not everyone adheres to such an approach, uninfected people must engage in primary prevention so that they do not contract HIV. For the infected person, enlightened self-interest demands preventing contact with a range of other sexually transmitted diseases, as well as HIV, either through sexual contact or by needle sharing. The danger of such contact is the potential for infection with other microorganisms that may have a deleterious impact on the primary HIV infection. Re-infection with HIV may result in HIV superinfection and the development of resistance to the medication regimen. This secondary prevention helps to maintain the health of the infected person. Tertiary prevention helps, for example, to maintain skin integrity by the use of lambskin and frequent turning to prevent the further deterioration of decubiti.

11. How long can an HIV-infected person expect to live?

The answer that "it depends" is not hedging. Some factors include the type of virus and its genetic make-up; the robustness of health of the host; the daily health maintenance activities of the host (e.g., sleep, nutrition); the expertise of the HIV health care provider; and ultimately some degree of luck. The average life expectancy is 11 years after HIV diagnosis. Obviously, those diagnosed later in the course of the illness may live for fewer years. Treatment, other factors being equal, is now withheld until the disease progresses. This recommendation is based on knowledge of currently available medications. The standard of care is likely to change if a new medication proves efficacious earlier in the disease process.

12. If medications are not available or desired, what then?

Medication therapy for people with HIV may not always be available or desirable. In many developing countries, antiretroviral therapy and other medications for HIV are limited. Some patients should not start medications because of potential problems with adherence to therapy. In addition, patients who experience side effects or other problems require adjustment and perhaps discontinuation of medications. In such circumstances, the nurse must continue to assess, monitor, intervene, and evaluate the patient's unique needs, focusing on maintaining health and preventing transmission of HIV. Before a decision is made that medications are not desired based on issues related to nonadherence, the nurse must consider strategies to improve adherence. The *Guidelines for the Use of Antiretroviral Agents in HIV-infected Adults and Adolescents* suggest the following strategies:

Strategies to Improve Adherence: Clinician- and Health Team-Related

- Establish trust.
- Serve as educator, source of information, ongoing support, and monitor.
- Provide access between visits for questions/problems via page number, including vacation/conference coverage.
- Monitor ongoing adherence; intensify management in periods of low adherence (i.e., more frequent visits, recruitment of family/friends, deployment of other team members, referral for mental health or chemical dependency services).
- Use health team for all patients, for difficult patients, for special needs (e.g., peer educators for adolescents or for injection drug users).
- Consider impact of new diagnoses on adherence (e.g., depression, liver disease, wasting, recurrent chemical dependency), and include adherence intervention in management.

Table continued on following page

Strategies to Improve Adherence: Clinician- and Health Team-Related (Continued)

• Use nurses, pharmacists, peer educators, volunteers, case managers, drug counselors, physician's assistants, nurse practitioners, and research nurses to reinforce message of adherence.

• Provide training to support team related to antiretroviral therapy and adherence.

• Add adherence interventions to job descriptions of HIV support team members; add continuity-of-care role to improve patient access (p. 39).

13. What are the components of palliative care for the person with HIV/AIDS?

The components of palliative care are the same for the person with HIV/AIDS and any other person with a potentially life-limiting disease. Examples include assiduous attention to physical symptoms, such as fatigue, peripheral neuropathy, and diarrhea. In addition to physical factors, attention is given to psychological, social, and spiritual factors. Financial issues are covered as part of social issues. The provision of palliative care does not imply cessation of treatment with antiretrovirals; rather, it indicates attention to symptoms that are most distressing to patients.

14. Is hospice care ever appropriate for someone who is HIV-infected?

Of course—as long as the patient has had access to a range of antiretroviral medications when they are generally available and is not choosing hospice care because of a lack of access to treatment. This statement, although applicable in the United State and other resource-rich societies, may not be applicable in resource-poor countries. In the U.S., patients do not have to choose between treatment and hospice care. Hospice programs now provide active treatment to HIV-infected patients. Nonetheless, some patients find that no effective treatment is available for them and that they are becoming increasingly weak and debilitated. Hospice care is appropriate for anyone with a life expectation of 6 months or less. Such an expectation is difficult for many patients and providers alike, and there is some discussion about the degree to which this criterion should be enforced.

15. What are the most significant health problems encountered by the person with HIV disease at different points in the illness trajectory?

The most significant health problems encountered by people with HIV include lymphadenopathy, respiratory problems (*Pneumocystis carinii* pneumonia, histoplasmosis, *Mycobacterium tuberculosis*), neurologic problems (toxoplasmosis, cryptococcal meningitis, lymphoma, cytomegalovirus), oral manifestations (candidiasis, oral hairy leukoplakia, herpes simplex virus, Kaposi's sarcoma, periodontitis), dermatologic manifestations (viral, fungal, bacterial, neoplastic, medication-related), liver problems (hepatitis and medication-related), pancreatic problems (often related to therapies), and gynecologic issues (candidiasis, human papillomavirus, cervical dysplasia, and cervical carcinoma).

16. What is the unique role of nursing in symptom management for people with HIV/ AIDS?

Nursing's unique role in symptom management is crucial to the health status and quality of life of the person living with HIV. Symptom management in HIV includes pharmacologic and nonpharmacologic interventions as well as complementary therapies than can be used for symptom control.

Pharmacologic measures can include a variety of medications directed at the underlying cause of the symptom or for comfort. For example, testosterone has been found to be helpful for a loss of libido in women as well as men. Leg pain due to a low vitamin B_{12} level can be addressed through supplementation. For cough due to tuberculosis, the underlying problem needs to be addressed, along with measures to prevent further transmission. Unfortunately, many of the problems that patients find most distressing are not readily amenable to pharmacologic management. Fatigue is a frequent complaint but is not adequately addressed by health care providers, in part because providers do not regard it as significant compared with other problems and in part because no therapy is readily available to resolve the problem. For this reason, patients often look to nonpharmacologic measures to resolve medical problems that interfere with their sense of well-being.

Nonpharmacologic measures may include nutrition, rest, exercise, and herbal preparations. Herbal medicines are of particular concern in that they may be used in place of medications with verified efficacy, depriving the patient of useful therapies. In addition, herbal preparations may interact with prescribed medications and either potentiate or lessen the effect. For example, St. John's wort has a negative interaction with ritonavir, one of the HAART medications. Worst of all, prescribed medications combined with street drugs have led to the deaths of users. The concern with the widespread use of herbal preparations and various other modalities that have not been tested rigorously for their efficacy has led to government-sponsored research to investigate these preparations. The initial impetus for funding such research was based on the belief that some of these approaches may be helpful to the user. The research will separate anecdotal from substantiated data.

Complementary therapies that can be helpful in symptom management include mind/body medicine techniques, alternative systems of medicine, and body work. Mind/body techniques are based on the interrelationship of the mind and body and the knowledge that patients can alleviate stress and other symptoms by calming the mind and facilitating healing. Some of the techniques used in mind/body healing include meditation, tai chi, qi gong, yoga, biofeedback, and guided imagery. Alternative systems of medicine include homeopathic medicine, Chinese medicine, Ayurvedic medicine, and acupuncture. Body work includes chiropractic therapies, therapeutic touch, massage therapy, reflexology, and qi gong. Further information may be obtained form the government website at www.nccam.nih.gov.

17. When should a person start antiretroviral therapy?

The HIV-positive person should start antiretroviral therapy when a thorough review of the history, physical exam, and laboratory diagnostic markers indicates that the patient is at risk for progression of disease. According to *The Guidelines for the Use of Antiretroviral Agents in HIV-infected Adults and Adolescents:*

> Evidence supports initiation of therapy in the asymptomatic HIV-infected person with a CD4+ T cell count < 350 cells/mm³ or a viral load > 55,000 copies/ml. For asymptomatic patients with a CD4+ T cell count > 350 cells/mm³, evidence supports both conservative and aggressive approaches to therapy. The **conservative approach** is based on the recognition that robust immune reconstitution still occurs in most patients who initiate therapy with CD4+ T cell counts in the range of 200–350 cells/mm³ and that toxicities and adherence challenges may outweigh benefits of initiating therapy at CD4+ T cell counts > 350 cells/mm³. In the conservative approach, high levels of plasma HIV RNA (i.e., > 55,000 by BDNA or RT-PCR) are an indication for more frequent monitoring of CD4+ T cell counts and plasma HIV RNA levels, but not necessarily for initiation of therapy. In the **aggressive approach**, asymptomatic patients with CD4+ T cell counts > 350 cells/mm³ and levels of plasma HIV RNA > 55,000 copies/ml are treated because of the risk of immunologic deterioration and disease progression. The aggressive approach is supported by the observation in many studies that suppression of plasma HIV RNA by antiretroviral therapy is easier to achieve and maintain at higher CD4+ T cell counts and lower levels of plasma viral load (pp. 8–9).

18. Whose responsibility is it to have safe sex?

From the previous discussion the answer to this question may be predicted: whoever is having sexual relations. As noted earlier, to prevent transmission, the HIV-infected person must use barriers if abstinence is not chosen. Furthermore, the law in some states requires that the HIV-infected person inform potential partners of his or her HIV status. This issue has been debated in some communities. There is no debate in the public health community that, unless two uninfected people are monogamous and mutually faithful, it is not safe to engage in unprotected sexual relations. In sum, it is everyone's responsibility to protect not only him- or herself but also sexual (and needle-sharing) partner(s).

19. When should a person consider discontinuing antiretroviral therapy?

The HIV-positive person should consider stopping antiretroviral therapy when adherence cannot be maintained, diagnostic markers indicate progression of HIV despite adjustments in medication therapy, or side effects severely affect the person's quality of life. The *Guidelines for the Use of Antiretroviral Agents in HIV-infected Adults and Adolescents* address considerations for continuing therapy. The guidelines suggest the following:

> As recommendations evolve, patients who have begun highly active antiretroviral therapy at CD4+ T cell counts > 350/mm^3 may wish to discontinue treatment. No clinical data address whether this should be done or can be accomplished safely. Potential benefits include reduction of toxicities, drug-drug interactions, selection of resistant variants, and improvement in the quality of life. Potential risks include rebound in viral replication and renewed immunologic deterioration. If the patient and clinician agree to discontinue therapy, the patient should be closely monitored (p. 9).

Before discontinuing therapy, specific guidelines for changing antiretroviral therapy for suspected drug failure should be considered. Discussion with the client about implications of changing versus discontinuing therapy and consultation with clinicians with considerable expertise in the care of HIV infected patients should be considered.

BIBLIOGRAPHY

U.S. Department of Health and Human Services and the H.J. Kaiser Foundation: Guidelines for the Use of Antiretroviral Agents in HIV-infected Adults and Adolescents. Washington, DC, 2002. Available at http://www.hivatis.org

6. TELEPHONE TRIAGE FOR PEOPLE WITH HIV/AIDS: YOU MAKE THE CALL

Yolanda Y. Wess, RN, BSN, *and Madeline Bronaugh,* RN, MSN, ACRN

Telephone triage is an important link to health care, especially for people infected with HIV. The care of people with HIV/AIDS is changing at an alarming rate with rapid improvements and advancements in medications and treatment protocols. Increased collaboration among the client, the community, and health care systems is a necessary component to ensure continuity of care and positive outcomes for the person infected with HIV/AIDS.

1. What is telephone triage?

It is the use of a telephone system to sort out patient concerns. Calls are placed by the patient or caregiver to the phone triage line to report symptoms or gain information. The nurse uses the information from the patient to assess the problem quickly and to advise the patient of possible choices of care. The phone system used may be basic or sophisticated, including a direct line or centralized phone center operation equipped with triage software to aid in decision-making. This chapter describes the phone line that is manned by the nurse, directly or indirectly by use of voice mail, without aid of sophisticated software to aid in decision-making. In either case, the use of the phone for triage of needs does not substitute for traditional face-to-face delivery of care; it serves as a complementary service to assist patients who otherwise may not receive care or who may choose the wrong level of care. Phone triage can operate after hours or as a service to aid delivery of care during normal business hours.

2. What are the goals of telephone triage in the outpatient setting for patients with HIV/AIDS?

Because a large number of HIV-infected patients inadequately use their medications, have difficulty with obtaining or keeping their appointments, and have insufficient support to manage the multiple symptoms and demands of HIV infection, multiple calls to the health care provider can result. Purposeful triage of these calls can be a benefit in the outpatient setting. Two primary goals of phone triage are as follows:

• To determine the priority of the patient's need
• To determine the appropriate level of and place for care.

Efficient delivery of care (clinic flow and use of staff) can be maintained with these two goals in the forefront. Patients with scheduled appointments can receive timely care, patients who call with an urgent can be worked into the schedule or receive a timely response, and patients who have emergency needs can be referred to the emergency department (ED) or other setting for the appropriate level of intervention. These goals provide high-quality care delivery to the HIV-infected patient with multiple needs, prevent costly ED visits, and encourage patient self-management and adherence, resulting in increased overall patient satisfaction.

3. What are the critical elements in the development of a telephone triage system?

• Training and skills development of staff
• Protocol development
• Development of documentation and assessment method

Without these three critical elements, care will be inconsistent, inefficient, or inappropriate. Their inclusion decreases liability for the nurse and the facility by producing an organized, consistent method for answering patient concerns.

4. What experience, skills or training are most helpful in assessing the needs of patients in telephone triage?

The interaction between the patient and the nurse that occurs over the phone is a unique caregiving interaction. Some may argue that phone triage is a "hands-off" approach to providing care or that it is not care at all. In fact, every interaction with the patient is meaningful and can add to the ability of the patient to manage his or her illness and adhere to treatment. The nurse who is able to make independent decisions, yet follow established protocols, is most suited for this type of interaction with patients. Good assessment skills, patience, and active listening are essential. Confidence in one's ability, with a minimum of two years of experience in multiple work settings, is helpful. An awareness of limitations in scope of practice is also helpful.

At a minimum, the training session must include decision-making method, use of protocols, basic triage principles, and documentation and communication skills.[3] Case studies, observation, and role-playing are highly recommended in the skill-building training session.[6] The nurse performing phone triage with HIV/AIDS patients must be knowledgeable of antiretroviral agents and their possible side effects. He or she must also be aware of the common symptoms of HIV disease and the basic terminology and pathophysiology of HIV disease.

5. What is the role of the nurse in telephone triage?

In telephone triage the nurse's role is varied. He or she is available to listen and assist the patient with navigating through multiple systems. For the patient infected with HIV/AIDS, the ability of the nurse to master this role plays an important part in whether positive outcomes are achieved. The nurse gathers information, makes a quick assessment of data, and determines priority of need. He or she functions as an advocate and resource by making choices available to the patient and facilitates access to care. He or she functions as a coordinator by scheduling appointments and assisting with arrangements for other services.

The nurse's role is not to diagnose or provide consultation, but to function as an advisor by following established protocols and directing patients to the most appropriate level and place of care. He or she is an educator, assisting the patient to understand instructions or treatments and asking for feedback if there is no improvement. In the role of caregiver, the nurse gives reassurance and encourages the patient to try interventions and to participate in care but allows the patient to make the final choice. A listing of available community resource phone numbers and addresses is an invaluable tool for the nurse to compile and use in acting in the role of resource to patients. The nurse is an integral member of the care team and should take advantage of ongoing opportunities to attend conferences about building skills in communication and assessment.

6. What are the critical components in the decision-making process for telephone triage?

In phone triage quick assessment of the need and ranking the priority of the need are the most critical decisions that must be made. The ranking of need is basically a determination of the required level of care. The need might be ranked as:

- **Emergent.** Symptoms ranked as an emergency need require immediate medical intervention and may cause a threat to life and/or functioning. The patient is instructed to call 911 or immediately go to the closest ED for evaluation.
- **Urgent.** Symptoms or concerns ranked as urgent require medical intervention within the next 24 hours but are not life-threatening. Patients are scheduled for an appointment on the same day or as the first appointment on the next day, if appropriate. Patients may also be directed to urgent care centers or other facilities, depending on the approved protocol.
- **Nonurgent.** Nonurgent symptoms or concerns are not emergent or acute. Patients are given advice or instructions according to protocol.

Once the assessment has been made, the level of care assigned, and the proper place of care determined, protocols are used to guide interventions and advice. The nurse should remember that brief, specific instructions are easier for a patient to follow than long explanations.[4] Evaluation is the final step of the decision-making process (see figure on following page).

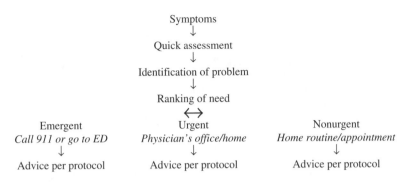

Symptoms
↓
Quick assessment
↓
Identification of problem
↓
Ranking of need
↔

Emergent	Urgent	Nonurgent
Call 911 or go to ED	*Physician's office/home*	*Home routine/appointment*
↓	↓	↓
Advice per protocol	Advice per protocol	Advice per protocol

Decision tree for telephone triage.

The nursing process is integral to nursing actions and is a good method to use for decision-making and problem-solving. The nursing process guides the nurse through the process of assessment, planning, intervention, and evaluation and reiterates the flow of decision-making suggested above. For example, decision-making for telephone nursing triage includes the following:

- Assessment: data collection, identification of problem, ranking of need.
- Planning: decision of which protocol to use.
- Intervention: advising the patient what to do.
- Evaluation: validation of understanding, patient outcomes, documentation.

7. What is a protocol? What information should be included in its development?

Protocols are established ways of managing patient needs and concerns. The development and consistent use of protocols are critical to successful telephone triage.[1] Protocols must be written. They guide care decisions by prompting assessment questions and assist in timely handling of needs. They provide a standardized approach for advice, instruction, and information sharing. When followed, they help to remove subjectivity and add consistency. In developing protocols the following components should be included:

- Identification of the problem
- Symptoms that characterize the problem
- Advice/intervention to be used to handle the problem
- Call-back instructions if the problem does not improve.

8. What are the most common concerns addressed during telephone triage with patients infected with HIV/AIDS?

A recent study[8] identified the following concerns as the most common reasons for telephone calls:

- I am out of refills.
- I have a rash since starting my HIV medications.
- I am tired all of the time since starting my HIV medications.
- I have no appetite.
- I have a fever that I can't get rid of.

9. How does HIV/AIDS telephone triage aid in patient self-management and adherence?

The nurse can use telephone triage as an excellent vehicle in identifying and promoting self-management and adherence. Adherence involves taking medications correctly, every day, and on time, all of the time. It has been identified as the single most important factor in treatment success for people with HIV/AIDS.[8] The professional nurse will use every opportunity that he or she has to promote the basic elements of self-management. HIV/AIDS telephone triage can identify a safe place for the client to connect with heath care. The client knows that his or her phone calls will be returned in a timely fashion, using the expertise of experienced HIV/AIDS nurses. A series of basic questions can be asked by the nurse as an adherence screen. The questions can be used as a framework in which to operate. The questions used on this screen are as follows:

1. Can you name your medications?
2. How do you take your medications?
3. Do you have difficulties from your medications that cause you to miss or skip a dose?

These questions can be answered with a simple yes or no and can be asked during the telephone triage process. The nurse can identify problematic areas for the client and provide valuable information, therefore increasing the knowledge base for the client and promoting self-management practices.

10. When is it time to consult the physician?

HIV/AIDS care should be based on the protocols established at your institution. Medically approved protocols, in accordance with the scope of practice for the professional nurse, establish a framework for care. Adhering to approved protocols enables you to identify situations in which medical consultation is appropriate. Each state has standards relating to competent practice as a registered nurse. Please refer to your nurse practice act and the rules and regulations of your state board of nursing in devising protocols. To assist you in the development of your protocols, refer to the figure on page 43. In addition, the nurse may want to provide the caller with the option to seek medical attention sooner if the caller does not agree with the advice.

11. Is a tracking system necessary?

Yes. Documentation of calls provides proof of consistency in approach and a record of the intervention/protocol used; it also assists in the evaluation of care and nursing performance. Much of the evaluation of quality occurs through chart audits of the documentation. Use of logs for calls returned to the patient aid in measuring patient outcomes. Each individual program should consider the need for collecting data about the number of calls received and the type of needs addressed during those calls. Good documentation acts as proof of provision of safe, standard care. Use of preprinted forms for documentation of the call is recommended. A typical note should include the following:

- Caller's name
- Patient's name
- Call-back phone number
- Date and time of call
- Patient's age
- Allergies
- Physician's name
- Symptoms reported
- Quick assessment by nurse
- Ranking of need
- Protocol/intervention used
- Advice given
- Patient's verbal response to advice

12. Does telephone triage increase patient satisfaction?

A telephone triage quality improvement survey may prove beneficial to substantiate the effectiveness of telephone triage. Some institutions may be involved with nationally recognized organizations (e.g., Press Ganey) for measuring patient satisfaction. However, each outpatient center may choose to devise a tool specifically to evaluate the needs of its institution. Immediate responses of satisfaction or dissatisfaction from patients are often received when the call is returned with recommendations. A call-log aids in collecting such responses. Routine review of surveys and logs can be used to measure satisfaction and improve care. Favorable outcomes that have been reported include decreased visits to the ED, improved rates of appointment keeping, and improved self-reported adherence and education.[2,3] An example of a telephone triage quality improvement survey is found on the following page.

Date and time of call _____
| | Yes | No |

1. Did the nurse respond promptly and adequately to your concerns?
2. Was the nurse courteous and professional?
3. Was the information received helpful?
4. Did you follow the instructions of the nurse?
5. Would you recommend our service to other people?

Comments:
_____
_____

Areas of improvement:
_____
_____

Follow-up needed?
Patient name: _____ Phone _____

Signature _____

Telephone triage patient satisfaction survey.

13. What are the legal constraints?

Many states have passed laws or have pending bills regarding medical care delivered across phone lines. There is even discussion of possible legislation to regulate care given over phone lines at the federal level. It is advisable to check with your local state legislature for any guidelines or restrictions. There are differences in how each state board of nursing defines the practice of nursing and the scope of practice of a nurse. Check with your local board for specific rules about how a nurse must practice in relation to care given over the phone. In all cases, there is a risk of liability with giving advice over the phone. Phone triage is limited by the inability to make a visual assessment of the patient. Standardization of care is one approach to limiting liability. Protocols and decision trees standardize decision-making and decrease error. Complete documentation of interactions is necessary to provide safe care and decrease liability. A few resources that provide specific information about rules governing telemedicine and telehealth are as follows:

- Telemedicine Research Center website: www.tie@telemed.org
- National Council of State Boards of Nursing website: www.ncsbn.org
- Federation of State Medical Boards website: www.fsmb.org

BIBLIOGRAPHY

1. Briggs JK: Telephone Triage Protocols for Nurses, 2nd ed. Philadelphia, J.B. Lippincott, 2002.
2. Chang BL: Consumer satisfaction with telehealth advice-nursing. Medinfo 10(Pt 2):1435–1439, 2001.
3. Greenberg ME: Telephone nursing: Evidence of client and organizational benefits. Nurs Econ 18(3):117–123, 2000.
4. Grossman VGA: Quick Reference to Triage. Philadelphia, J.B. Lippincott, 1999.
5. Infectious Disease Center, University of Cincinnati, Health Alliance: Interview of Nursing Staff about Telephone Triage. Infectious Disease Center, University of Cincinnati, Health Alliance, Cincinnati, OH, June 2000.
6. Katz HP: Telephone Medicine: Triage and Training for Primary Care, 2nd ed. Philadelphia, F. A. Davis, 2001.
7. Simonsen SM: Telephone Health Assessment: Guidelines for Practice, 2nd ed. St. Louis, Mosby, 2001.
8. Stone VE, Hogan JW, Schuman P, et al: Antiretroviral regimen complexity, self-reported adherence, and HIV patients' understanding of their regimens: A survey of women in the HER study. J Acq Immune Defic Syndr 28:124–132, 2001.

7. COMPLEMENTARY THERAPIES

Kenneth Zwolski, RN, EdD, FNP-CS

In the United States, most types of health treatments, approaches, and philosophies that do not fit within the paradigm of traditional Western medicine are collectively referred to as either alternative or complementary medicine. Today the two terms are usually combined into one: complementary alternative medicine (CAM).

1. What is meant by the term *CAM*?

CAM embraces a wide spectrum of health care approaches, ranging from self-care according to folk principles to care rendered in an organized health care setting. Ayurveda (see question 10), traditional Chinese medicine (see question 11), and Tibetan medicine are traditional non-Western systems that factor heavily into CAM approaches and are characterized by the use of many modalities, including acupuncture, meditation, acupressure, yoga, herbs, breathing and relaxation techniques, dietary systems, and movement therapy, such as tai chi and qi qong. Other CAM modalities include vitamin therapy, manual healing techniques, massage, visualization and imagery, aerobic and anaerobic exercise, and aromatherpay. Any integrative mind/body approach other than Western medicine can be considered CAM. Prayer and spirituality are considered by many clients to be integral parts of any CAM approach. CAM places great importance on assessing and treating the whole person. The Food and Drug Administration (FDA) often does not approve CAM treatments. Third-party payers, such as insurance companies, do not reimburse for many CAM treatments.

2. Why is the term *CAM* preferable to the term *alternative therapies*?

The term *alternative* is now infrequently used by itself for two reasons. First, what is alternative in one culture may be mainstream in another culture (e.g., acupuncture). Second, therapies that are used outside the mainstream of traditional Western medicine are often used to complement traditional approaches. They are not used to replace them or to substitute for them as the term *alternative* implies.

3. Do any statistics or studies indicate how many people use complementary therapies?

In 1993 Eisenberg and colleagues[2] published the results of one of the first studies to focus on the use of complementary therapies by people in the United States. They showed that CAM was used extensively in this country. In addition, they found that most people used CAM in a truly complementary fashion; that is, 83% of people using CAM for serious medical conditions also sought help from physicians. One startling finding from this study, however, was that 75% of people using CAM did not inform their traditional Western provider.

4. How many people with HIV/AIDS use complementary therapy?

Sparber et al.[6] randomly sampled 100 patients diagnosed with HIV who were receiving treatment either at the National Cancer Institute or the National Institutes of Allergy and Infectious Disease. They found that 91% had used at least one CAM therapy at some time in their life. After receiving their diagnosis of HIV/AIDS, 84% had used at least one CAM therapy. Singh et al.[5] found that 30–50% of clients with HIV have tried some form of complementary therapy.

5. Why do people with HIV/AIDS seek and use complementary therapies?

In the study by Sparber et al.,[6] people using CAM reported the following benefits:
- Increased coping ability (100%)
- Feeling better (98.1%)

• Enhanced treatment outcomes (94.2%). Most (61%) reported that CAM was more success-ful for them than regular treatment.
• Feeling in control (88.5%)

In another study, Cain and Gillett[1] reported results of 66 people with HIV who had used or were using complementary therapies. These complementary therapies represented different things to different people: a health maintenance strategy, a healing strategy, an alternative to Western medicine, a way for mitigating the side effects of drug therapies, a strategy for maximiz-ing the quality of life, a coping strategy, or a form of political resistance. The meaning given to complementary therapies and the expected benefits were linked to sexuality; ethnocultural back-ground; gender; beliefs about health and illness; and personal values and experiences. The over-riding conclusion was that complementary therapies appeal to people at different levels. In general, clients with HIV/AIDS use CAM for the following purposes:

• Because of the paucity of consistently effective therapies for managing symptoms
• As a search for meaning
• As an attempt to strengthen the body's resistance
• As a counter for the side effects of medication
• As a reduction of stress.

6. What complementary therapies are being used?

The list of therapies, in order of popularity, is continually changing and growing. The fol-lowing table summarizes the most frequently used CAM modalities among people with HIV/AIDS, according to results from recent studies.

Most Frequently Used CAM Modalities

ACCORDING TO SPARBER AT AL.[6]	ACCORDING TO GREENE ET AL.[3]
Imagery	Aerobic exercises (64%)
High-dose vitamins	Prayer (56%)
Weight gain	Massage (54%)
Massage	Needle acupuncture (48%)
Relaxation	Meditation (46%)
Herbals	Support groups (42%)
Spiritual activities	Visualization and imagery (34%)
Acupuncture	Breathing exercises (33%)
	Spiritual activities (33%)
	Other exercises (33%)

7. How do complementary therapies fit into the overall treatment of people with HIV/AIDS?

The overall goal of CAM is to design the best combination treatment available for a person with HIV. With the widespread use of antiretroviral therapy, CAM can be used to reduce the severity of side effects and to treat conditions that do not respond well to antiretroviral therapy (e.g., wasting syndrome). CAM provides individualization of care not often available with other therapies.

8. Are vitamins considered a complementary therapy?

Yes. Clients with HIV/AIDS frequently use vitamins and minerals, often in unconventional doses. They take vitamins for a variety of reasons; for example, to replace levels of vitamins de-creased due to the disease process itself, to increase the amount of vitamins in the body above normal levels, and to counter symptoms of HIV/AIDS.

The disease process itself may decrease the level of vitamins available in the body, increase the need for vitamins, or both. Hence, it is difficult to determine the exact amount of vitamins that a client with HIV/AIDS needs. There is little danger of toxicity from large doses of water-soluble vitamins, but the fat-soluble vitamins (A, D, E and K) can be retained in the body for a long period. Therefore, any client taking megadoses of these vitamins should be monitored.

Clients often take vitamins to treat fatigue, weight loss, nerve pain, and muscle cramps. Antioxidants have been shown to protect against free radicals. In this sense, they may offer some degree of protection to the immune system. Among the vitamins, C and E are antioxidants. Tang's study[7] showed that HIV clients who had the highest levels of vitamin E had a 34% reduction in the risk of disease progression compared with those with the lowest levels of vitamin E. It is not clear whether the higher level of vitamin E was responsible for the slowed disease progression or vice versa. In addition, factors other than the vitamin may have contributed to slowed disease progression.

9. What herbs are used most commonly to treat people with HIV/AIDS?

- Echinacea: thought to increase immune system functioning by stimulating T cells (although stimulation of T cells may not be in the best interest of a client with HIV/AIDS, because it may lead to the increased replication of the virus)
- Garlic: thought to have antibacterial and antiviral properties
- Hyssop: applied externally as an ointment; may be used in the treatment of Kaposi's sarcoma
- St. John's wort: noted for its antidepressant effects; may have broad-spectrum antiviral activity

In addition, clients being treated within the framework of traditional Chinese medicine may avail themselves of numerous Chinese herbs that are thought to enhance the immune system, including astralagus, ganoderma, Asian ginseng, and licorice. Three popular herbal formulas (compounds of several herbs) are called Resist, Clear Heat, and Enhance.

10. What is Ayurveda?

Ayurveda is ancient yet modern. It originated on the Indian subcontinent over 3,000 years ago and continues to be influenced by modern science. Ayurveda is a system of achieving and maintaining health. Health, however, is not considered the final goal but rather as an important condition for spiritual growth.[8] According to Ayurveda, the cosmos is composed of five basic elements or mahabatus: earth, air, fire, water, and space. In living matter these five elements come together and give rise to the fundamental physiologic energy that regulates the body. This energy is called the dosha. Three doshas can occur: vata, pitta, and kapha. A person is usually a combination of two of these doshas. To maintain good health, a person must keep his or her doshas in balance.

Several factors other than doshas must be considered in assessing a person's health, including dhatus (tissues), malas (waste), srotas (the channels through which substances circulate), and agnis (digestive enzymes). Digestion is considered by Ayurveda to be one of the most important functions to take place in the human body; when it is not working, undigested food (ama) results. Ama is a principal cause of maladies.

Ayurvedic treatment is both prophylactic (i.e., maintaining a normal condition) and therapeutic. Treatment may include purification through sweating, use of purgatives or enemas, and use of herbs and foods characterized on the basis of their innate qualities. The emphasis in Ayurveda is on maintaining a healthy state. Many regimens are recommended to achieve this goal. Typical regimens include meditation, proper diet, periodic fasting, aromatherapy, self-massage, the use of oil, and regularity in daily routines.

11. What is traditional Chinese medicine?

Traditional Chinese medicine (TCM) is a system that focuses on the whole person. The concept of qi is at the core of TCM. Qi , the universal energy that runs through each person, flows through well-defined meridians or channels within the body. The terms *yin* and *yang* are used to describe the location, movement, function, and quality of the qi. Yin and yang are opposites. Yin is passive, internal, cold, and feminine in nature. Yang is active, external, hot, and masculine in nature. Disease is seen as a disharmony or imbalance between yin and yang. The imbalance can cause qi to become excessive or deficient. The disharmony can also result when qi becomes stagnant.

Therapies in TCM are directed at restoring harmony, promoting balance, and mobilizing stagnant qi. Herbs, which are characterized by their inherent properties, can be prescribed to remedy a yin or yang excess or deficit. Acupuncture, through the manipulation of meridians, can unblock stagnant qi. Qi qong combines aerobic, isometric, and isotonic exercise with the relaxation response, meditation, and guided imagery to keep qi flowing and balanced.

12. Are any known dangers associated with the use of complementary therapies?

Providers must remember that many CAM treatments have not been rigorously tested. One possible complication of high-dose micronutrient therapy is gastrointestinal distress, along with other nutrient-specific side effects. Little conclusive evidence indicates that extremely high doses of vitamins and minerals have beneficial effects. In some cases, megadoses of minerals may be detrimental. For example, megadoses of zinc can lead to impaired immune function along with gastrointestinal distress. Megadoses of calcium can lead to constipation and impaired kidney function.

Herbs need to be monitored. The Centers for Disease Control and Prevention (CDC) have reported deaths associated with the use of ephedrine or mahuang, an herb found in various teas and herbal formulations. Certain herbs, including chaparral, germander, comfrey, mistletoe, skullcap, margosa oil, gordoloba yerba tea, pennyroyal (squawmint oil), and some types of Mate teas, have also been associated with toxicity and even death. Kobucha is a Manchurian mushroom, taken as a tea, that has attained a certain degree of popularity. However, people with HIV should be advised that other disease-producing organisms, such as *Aspergillus* species, may grow in the brew; they may be dangerous for people with a suppressed immune system. Likewise, shark cartilage, which is used by many people with HIV/AIDS, smells foul, is difficult to take orally, causes nausea and vomiting, and is poorly absorbed by the stomach.

Patients taking antiretroviral drugs must know that many herbs and vitamins, like many anti-HIV drugs, are metabolized by the liver and excreted by the kidneys. Powerful drug-herb interactions can occur. Pregnant women with HIV have additional concerns that need to be addressed and followed in close consultation with the primary care provider and obstetrician.

Piscatelli et al.[4] found that St. John's wort can reduce the blood levels of indinavir, a protease inhibitor that is an important part of many antiretroviral drug regimens. Such reductions may interfere with the efficacy of the drug, and people who take indinavir should be advised not to take St. John's wort at the same time.

13. How do you evaluate the effectiveness of complementary therapies?

The basic concepts of safety and efficacy need to be evaluated in determining the effectiveness of complementary therapies. Some tips to share with clients in their efforts to choose reputable and effective therapies include the following:

- Look for published studies in reputable journals.
- Be wary of personal testimonials; be alert for fraud or claims about miracles or cures.
- Know what ingredients are used; secret ingredients should be deemed unacceptable.
- Be skeptical of treatments that promise to cure several illnesses.
- Be wary of any treatment that requires discontinuing other components of a regular regimen.
- Carefully examine reports conducted in developing countries, where standards and procedures may differ.

14. How should a client talk to the health care practitioner about the use of complementary therapies?

Communication must be improved between the traditional health care provider and the client who is either interested in CAM or already using CAM modalities. It is also important to be able to communicate effectively with CAM practitioners and to choose the correct CAM provider for the situation. Below are some tips for helping clients discuss complementary therapies with their primary provider or their CAM provider and to make decisions about the choice of a CAM provider:

- Describe your symptoms completely.
- Keep a symptom diary.
- If you are interested in CAM, ask what the primary care practitioner knows about it and request assistance in finding a qualified CAM practitioner.
- Once you identify a CAM practitioner, interview him or her, ask of what the treatment will consist, what it will cost, when results should appear, what are the likely side effects, and whether third-party reimbursement is available.
- Ask if the CAM practitioner is willing to speak with your primary care provider about treatment recommendations and side effects and to forward your records.
- Ask if it is possible to speak to other patients treated by the CAM provider.
- Look for legitimate CAM practitioners. Many are licensed, such as naturopathic physicians, acupuncturists, practitioners of Chinese medicine, massage therapists, and hypnotherapists.
- Consult with local and state medical boards, other health regulatory boards or agencies, and consumer affairs departments, all of which may be sources of information about a practitioner's education and license and whether any complaints have been filed against that person.
- [a] Ask the practitioner directly about his or her training, education, and license.
- Evaluate the practitioner's willingness to communicate about technical aspects and benefits or risks.
- Visit the provider's office or clinic to observe the quality of service.

15. How much do nurses need to know about complementary therapies?

Nurses need to develop a way to acknowledge and potentially incorporate CAM into HIV disease management. A significant portion of people with HIV use CAM, and many do not talk about it with their health care providers. Nurses need to recognize that patients use CAM and become acquainted with and conversant about CAM options. Encourage the patient to keep a symptom diary as a means of helping to evaluate and monitor the use of CAM. Convey a positive and accepting attitude. Try to integrate CAM into the client's daily regimens and routines. Always keep in mind that CAM allows many patients to take a more active role in their care and thus can empower them.

BIBLIOGRAPHY

1. Cain D, Gillett J: Lay construction of HIV and complementary therapy use. Soc Sci Med 2000 51:251–264, 2000.
2. Eisenberg DM, et al: Unconventional medicine in the United States: Prevalence, costs and patterns of use. N Engl J Med 328(4):246, 1993.
3. Greene KB, et al: Most frequently used alternative and complementary therapies and activities by participants in the AMCOA study. JANAC 10(3): 60–73, 1999.
4. Piscatelli SC, et al: Indinavir concentration and St. John's wort. Lancet 335:547, 2000.
5. Singh N, et al: Determinants fo nontraditional therapy use in patients with HIV infection. Arch Intern Med 156(2):197, 1996.
6. Sparber A, et al: Use of complementary medicine by adult patients participating in HIV/AIDS clinical trials. Altern Complement Med 6:415–422, 2000.
7. Tang A: Vitamin E slows AIDS progression. AIDS 11:613, 1995.
8. Zwolski K: Ayurveda. In Clark CC (ed): The Encyclopedia of Complementary Health Practices. New York, Springer Publishing, 1999.

8. POSTEXPOSURE PROPHYLAXIS

Lyn Stevens, MS, ACRN, NP

You are at work, and a needle punctures your hand. Do you know what to do next? HIV infection may be transmitted through accidental exposure in the health care setting. Prompt initiation of prophylaxis is recommended for exposed workers. Joint Centers for Disease Control and Prevention (CDC) and Public Health Service guidelines for determining the need for prophylaxis are based on assessing the risk of transmission and the HIV status of the exposure source.[7] Every health care worker must know his or her agency's policy and procedure regarding postexposure prophylaxis. If you are unaware of the policy, become informed and encourage coworkers to learn it.

1. What is the risk of HIV transmission through occupational exposure?

In prospective studies of health care workers, the average risk of HIV transmission after a percutaneous exposure to HIV-infected blood has been estimated to be approximately 0.3% and after mucous membrane exposure, approximately 0.09%. Although episodes of HIV transmission after nonintact skin exposure have been documented, the average risk for transmission by this route has not been precisely quantified but is estimated to be less than the risk for mucous membrane exposures. The risk for transmission after exposure to fluids or tissues other than HIV-infected blood also has not been quantified but is probably considerably lower than for blood exposures.[3]

Studies suggest that several factors may affect the risk of HIV transmission after an occupational exposure. In a retrospective, case-controlled study of health care workers with percutaneous exposure to HIV, the risk for HIV infection was found to be increased with exposure to a larger quantity of blood from the source person. Other factors include the following:

- Device visibly contaminated with the patient's blood
- Procedure that involved placement of a needle directly in a vein or artery
- Deep injury
- Terminal illness of the source patient (possibly reflecting a higher titer of HIV in the blood)

As of June 2000, the CDC had received voluntary reports of 56 U.S. health care workers with documented HIV seroconversion thought to be associated with an occupational exposure. An additional 138 episodes in health care workers are considered possible occupational HIV transmissions. These workers had a history of occupational exposure to blood, other infectious body fluids, or laboratory solutions containing HIV. No other risk for HIV infection was identified, but HIV seroconversion after a specific event was not documented.

2. What is postexposure prophylaxis (PEP)?

PEP refers to using a combination of certain drugs called antiretrovirals to reduce the risk of HIV infection for health care workers after exposure to the blood or body fluids of a patient with HIV.

3. Does PEP work?

Several clinical studies have demonstrated that HIV transmission can be significantly reduced by the administration of antiretroviral agents. In a retrospective, case-controlled study of health care workers, the CDC showed that, after controlling for other risk factors for HIV transmission, use of zidovudine (AZT) for PEP was associated with a reduction in the risk of HIV infection by approximately 81%.[2] The AIDS Clinical Trials Group (ACTG) protocol 076 was a multicenter trial in which AZT was administered to HIV-infected pregnant women and their infants. The administration of AZT during pregnancy, labor, and delivery and to the infant reduced transmission by 67%.

Although these findings support the potential benefits of PEP, approximately 22 failures have been documented worldwide.[4] Factors that contribute to PEP failure are exposure to large viral inoculum (substance containing HIV), delayed initiation of antiretroviral therapy, use of AZT monotherapy, and exposure to drug-resistant virus.

4. What should you do if you have an exposure?

1. *Provide care to the exposure site immediately.* Cleanse the wound and skin sites with soap and water. Flush exposed mucous membranes with water. Do not use chemicals that will cause irritation (e.g., bleach), and do not "milk" the site to make it bleed. Both actions cause inflammation at the site and are not recommended.

2. *Speak with your supervisor to determine the risk associated with exposure.* Consider the type of fluid and the type of exposure, infectious status of source, and susceptibility of the exposed person. The CDC recommendations for assessment of exposure are listed in the tables below.

Recommended HIV Postexposure Prophylaxis (PEP) for Percutaneous Injuries[3]

	INFECTION STATUS OF SOURCE				
EXPOSURE TYPE	HIV-POSITIVE CLASS 1*	HIV-POSITIVE CLASS 2*	UNKNOWN HIV STATUS[†]	UNKNOWN SOURCE[‡]	HIV-NEGATIVE
Less severe[§]	Recommend basic 2-drug PEP	Recommend expanded 3-drug PEP	Generally, no PEP warranted; but consider basic 2-drug PEP[¶] for source with HIV risk factors[//]	Generally, no PEP warranted; but consider basic 2-drug PEP[¶] in settings where exposure to HIV-infected persons is likely	No PEP warranted
More severe[∞]	Recommend expanded 3-drug PEP	Recommend expanded 3-drug PEP	Generally, no PEP warranted; but consider basic 2-drug PEP[¶] for source with HIV risk factors	Generally, no PEP warranted but consider basic 2-drug PEP[¶] in settings where exposure to HIV-infected persons is likely	No PEP warranted

* HIV-positive, Class 1: asymptomatic HIV infection or known low viral load (e.g., < 1500 RNA copies/ml). HIV-positive, Class 2: symptomatic HIV infection, AIDS, acute seroconversion, or known high viral load. If drug resistance is a concern, obtain expert consultation. Initiation of PEP should not be delayed pending expert consultation, and, because expert consultation alone cannot substitute for face-to-face counseling, resources should be available to provide immediate evaluation and follow-up care for all exposures.
† Source of unknown HIV status (e.g., deceased person with no samples available for HIV testing).
‡ Unknown source (e.g.,.a needle from a sharps disposal container).
§ Less severe (e.g., solid needle and superficial injury).
¶ The designation "Consider PEP" indicates that PEP is optional and should be based on an individual decision between the exposed person and treating clinician.
// If PEP is offered and taken and the source is later determined to be HIV-negative, PEP should be discontinued.
∞ More severe (e.g., large-bore hollow needle, deep puncture, visible blood on device, or needle used in patient's artery or vein).

Recommended HIV PEP for Mucous Membrane Exposures and Nonintact Skin* Exposures[3]

	INFECTION STATUS OF SOURCE				
EXPOSURE TYPE	HIV-POSITIVE CLASS 1[†]	HIV-POSITIVE CLASS 2[†]	UNKNOWN HIV STATUS[‡]	UNKNOWN SOURCE[§]	HIV-NEGATIVE
Small volume[¶]	Consider basic 2-drug PEP[//]	Recommend basic 2-drug PEP	Generally, no PEP warranted; but consider basic 2-drug PEP[//] for source with HIV risk factors[∞]	Generally, no PEP warranted; but consider basic 2-drug PEP[//] in settings where exposure to HIV-infected persons is likely	No PEP warranted

Table continued on following page

Recommended HIV PEP for Mucous Membrane Exposure and Nonintact Skin* Exposures (Continued)

EXPOSURE TYPE	INFECTION STATUS OF SOURCE				
	HIV-POSITIVE CLASS 1[†]	HIV-POSITIVE CLASS 2[†]	UNKNOWN HIV STATUS[‡]	UNKNOWN SOURCE[§]	HIV-NEGATIVE
Large volume[#]	Recommend basic 2-drug PEP[//]	Recommend expanded 3-drug PEP	Generally, no PEP warranted; but consider basic 2-drug PEP[//] for source with HIV risk factors[∞]	Generally, no PEP warranted; but consider basic 2-drug PEP[//] in settings where exposure to HIV-infected persons is likely	No PEP warranted

* For skin exposures, follow-up is indicated only with evidence of compromised skin integrity (e.g., dermatitis, abrasion, or open wound).
[†] HIV-positive, Class 1: asymptomatic HIV infection or known low viral load (e.g., < 1500 RNA copies/ml). HIV-positive, Class 2: symptomatic HIV infection, AIDS, acute seroconversion, or known high viral load. If drug resistance is a concern, obtain expert consultation. Initiation of PEP should not be delayed pending expert consultation, and, because expert consultation alone cannot substitute for face-to-face counseling, resources should be available to provide immediate evaluation and follow-up care for all exposures.
[‡] Source of unknown HIV status (e.g., deceased person with no samples available for HIV testing).
[§] Unknown source (e.g,. splash from inappropriately disposed blood).
[¶] Small volume (i.e., a few drops).
[//] The designation, "Consider PEP," indicates that PEP is optional and should be based on an individual decision between the exposed person and treating clinician.
[∞] If PEP is offered and taken and the source is later determined to be HIV-negative, PEP should be discontinued.
[#] Large volume (i.e., major blood splash).

3. *Document.* After an occupational exposure, record the following information in the health care worker's confidential medical record: date and time of the exposure; details of the procedure being performed and the use of protective equipment at the time of the exposure; the type, severity, and amount of fluid to which the health care worker was exposed; details about the exposure source; and medical documentation that provides details about postexposure management.

4. *Evaluate exposure source.* If the source is known, determine HIV status. Assess HIV-positive sources for current viral load, CD4 count, and current and past medications. Encourage a patient of unknown HIV status to be tested for HIV, hepatitis B, and hepatitis C. If the source is unknown, assess the risk of exposure.

5. *Receive medical care.* Seek care as soon as possible, ideally 1–2 hours after exposure but definitely within 24 hours. Follow employer policy for where to receive such care. Many policies suggest going to the employee health office or the nearest emergency department. In some instances, the agency's medical director determines whether it is appropriate to initiate PEP. If a recommendation is made to begin PEP and the health care worker declines, this decision should be documented in the worker's medical record. Some agencies have the health care worker sign a statement that the recommendation was made and refused.

6. *Evaluate the exposed person.* Assess HIV status and immune status for hepatitis B and C.

7. *Prescribe PEP.* Decide whether PEP will be provided based on exposure and source patient information.

8. *Participate in follow-up care* (see discussion in question 7).

5. How do you determine whether the exposure is "significant"?

Postexposure treatment is not recommended for all occupational exposures to HIV because most exposures do not lead to HIV infection and the drugs used to prevent infection may have serious side effects. The tables in question 4 list recommendations that apply to situations in which a person has been exposed to a source with HIV infection or in which information suggests the likelihood that the source is HIV-infected. These recommendations are based on the risk for HIV infection after different types of exposure and on limited data regarding efficacy and toxicity of PEP.[3]

New York State has published guidelines that offer a simplified approach to assessment of significance. The guidelines state that PEP is indicated if the health care worker meets one or more of the following criteria:

- Break in the skin by a sharp object (including both hollow-bore and cutting needles or broken glassware) that is contaminated with blood, visibly bloody fluid, or other potentially infectious material or that has been in the patient's blood vessel
- Bite from an HIV-infected patient with visible bleeding in the mouth that causes bleeding in the health care worker
- Splash of blood, visibly bloody fluid, or other potentially infectious material to a mucosal surface (mouth, nose, or eyes)
- Nonintact skin (e.g., dermatitis, chapped skin, abrasion, or open wound) exposed to blood, visibly bloody fluid, or other potentially infectious material

It is important to check with your own state governing agency to determine guidelines for your specific area.

6. What medications are recommended?

The Public Health Service recommends a 4-week course of two drugs (AZT and lamivudine [Epivir, 3TC]) for most HIV exposures or AZT and lamivudine plus a protease inhibitor (indinavir [Crixivan] or nelfinavir [Viracept]) for exposures that may pose a greater risk for transmitting HIV (such as those involving a larger volume of blood with a larger amount of HIV or concern about drug-resistant HIV). Differences in side effects associated with the use of these two protease inhibitors may influence which drug is selected in a specific situation. These recommendations are intended to provide guidance to clinicians and may be modified on a case-by-case basis. Whenever possible, consulting an expert with experience in the use of antiviral drugs is advised.

Treatment should be started promptly, preferably within hours, as opposed to days, after exposure. Although animal studies suggest that treatment is not effective when started more than 24–36 hours after exposure, it is not known whether the same time frame applies to humans. Starting treatment after a longer period may be considered for the highest-risk exposures; even if HIV infection is not prevented, early treatment of initial HIV infection may lessen the severity of symptoms and delay the onset of AIDS.

Public Health Service Suggested Regimens[3]

BASIC REGIMEN	EXPANDED REGIMEN
Zidovudine, 300 mg twice daily	Basic 2-drug regimen *plus* one of the following:
Lamivudine, 150 mg twice daily *or* Combivir, 1 tablet twice daily (combination of AZT and 3TC)	Indinavir, 800 mg every 8 hr on an empty stomach Nelfinavir, 1250 mg twice daily with meals or snacks Efavirenz, 600 mg/day at bedtime

New York State recommends the use of three antiretrovirals in all instances of PEP. Any variance from this recommendation should be made in consultation with an HIV specialist.

Once the decision is made to offer PEP, the health care worker must be informed of the potential benefits and limitations of these medications.

7. Now that PEP is started, what next?

Discuss medical follow-up:

- HIV antibody testing: baseline, 6 weeks, 12 weeks, 6 months
- Complete blood count, kidney, and liver function tests: baseline, 2 weeks after treatment is started
- Pregnancy test, if appropriate
- Symptom reporting: sudden or severe flu-like illness that occurs during the follow-up period, especially if it involves fever, rash, muscle aches, tiredness, malaise, or swollen glands. Any of these may suggest HIV infection, drug reaction, or other medical conditions.

- Adherence support
- Side effect management
- Secondary prevention. During the first 6–12 weeks when most infected people are expected to show signs of infection, the health care worker should follow recommendations for preventing transmission of HIV: avoidance of donating blood, semen, or organs and avoidance of sexual intercourse. If the worker has sexual intercourse, consistent and correct use of a condom may reduce the risk of HIV transmission. In addition, women should consider not breast-feeding infants during the follow-up period to prevent exposure to HIV in breast milk.

8. What should be done when the health care worker says, "These meds are making me sick"?

The most common side effects associated with the antiretrovirals prescribed for PEP are nausea (58%), fatigue (38%), headache (18%), vomiting (16%), and diarrhea(14%).[9] The following table includes the most common drugs and side effects. Side effects are generally self-limited but may result in discontinuation of PEP in 20– 50% of health care workers.[7] The clinician prescribing PEP must discuss possible side effects and their management when PEP is initiated. Encourage the health care worker not to stop the medication without speaking to the clinician first.

Taking the medications as prescribed is vital to facilitate absorption and to prevent resistance. Medication sheets that explain how to take the drugs, possible side effects and their management strategies, and a number to call if clients have questions or concerns about treatment should be a part of counseling.

Primary Side Effects Associated with Antiretroviral Agents[3]

ANTIRETROVIRAL AGENT	PRIMARY SIDE EFFECTS AND TOXICITIES
Nucleoside reverse transcriptase inhibitors (NRTIs)	
Zidovudine (Retrovir; ZDV, AZT)	Anemia, neutropenia, nausea, headache, insomnia, muscle pain, and weakness
Lamivudine (Epivir; 3TC)	Abdominal pain, nausea, diarrhea, rash, and pancreatitis
Nonnucleoside reverse transcriptase inhibitor (NNRTI)	
Efavirenz (Sustiva; EFV)	Rash (including cases of Stevens-Johnson syndrome), insomnia, somnolence, dizziness, trouble concentrating, and abnormal dreaming
Protease inhibitors (PIs)	
Indinavir (Crixivan; IDV)	Nausea, abdominal pain, nephrolithiasis, and indirect hyperbilirubinemia
Nelfinavir (Viracept; NFV)	Diarrhea, nausea, abdominal pain, weakness, and rash

9. What are the risks of occupational exposure to hepatitis B and hepatitis C?

Approximately 800 health care workers become infected with the **hepatitis B virus** (HBV) each year after an occupational exposure. Risk from a single needlestick or cut exposure to HBV-infected blood ranges from 6% to 30%, depending on the hepatitis B e antigen (HBeAg) status of the source person. People who test positive for both hepatitis B surface antigen (HBsAg) and HBeAg have more virus in their blood and are more likely to transmit HBV.

There are no sound estimates of the number of health care workers occupationally infected with the **hepatitis C virus** (HCV). However, studies have shown that 1% of hospital health care workers have evidence of HCV infection. The number of workers who may have been infected through occupational exposure is unknown. The risk for infection after a needlestick or cut exposure to HCV-infected blood is approximately 1.8%. The risk following a blood splash is unknown but is believed to be very small. However, HCV infection from such an exposure has been reported.

10. How is occupational exposure to HBV managed?

The hepatitis B vaccine has been available since 1982 to prevent HBV infection. All health care workers who have a reasonable chance of exposure to blood or body fluids should receive hepatitis B vaccine. Workers should be tested 1–2 months after the vaccine series to make sure that vaccination has provided immunity to HBV infection. This vaccine is very safe. No information indicates that the vaccine causes any chronic illnesses.

Hepatitis B immune globulin (HBIG) is effective in preventing HBV infection after an exposure. The decision to begin treatment is based on several factors, such as whether the source person is positive for hepatitis B surface antigen, whether the health care worker has been vaccinated, and whether the vaccine provided immunity. When exposure occurs in a worker who has not been vaccinated, hepatitis B vaccination is recommended, regardless of the source person's hepatitis B status. HBIG and/or hepatitis B vaccine may be recommended, depending on the worker's immunity to hepatitis B and the source person's infection status. Treatment should begin as soon as possible after exposure, preferably within 24 hours and no later than 7 days.

Routine follow-up after HBV exposure is not recommended because PEP is highly effective. However, any symptoms suggesting hepatitis (yellow skin or eyes, loss of appetite, nausea, vomiting, fever, stomach or joint pain, extreme tiredness) should be reported.

11. How is occupational exposure to HCV managed?

There is no vaccine against hepatitis C, and no treatment after an exposure will prevent infection. Immune globulin is not recommended. Follow-up should include an antibody test for HCV and a liver enzyme test as soon as possible after the exposure (baseline) and at 4–6 months later. Some clinicians may also recommend another test (HCV RNA) to detect HCV infection 4–6 weeks after the exposure. Review with the worker the symptoms of HCV and the need to report to the health care provider if any of these symptoms develop.

12. Who pays for the medication and medical follow-up?

The employer of personnel covered by the *Occupational Safety and Health Administration (OSHA) Bloodborne Pathogen Standard* is obligated to provide postexposure care, including prophylaxis, at no cost to the employee. The employer may subsequently attempt to obtain reimbursement from Workers' Compensation.

13. Should all agencies have a PEP policy and procedure?

Health care organizations should make available to their personnel a system that includes written protocols for prompt reporting, evaluation, counseling, treatment, and follow-up of occupational exposures that may place a worker at risk for acquiring a bloodborne infection. Health care workers should be educated about the risk for and prevention of bloodborne infections, including the need to be vaccinated against hepatitis B. Employers are required to establish exposure-control plans that include postexposure follow-up for their employees and to comply with incident-reporting requirements mandated by the 1991 OSHA bloodborne pathogen standard. Access to clinicians who can provide postexposure care should be available during all working hours, including nights and weekends. HBIG, hepatitis B vaccine, and antiretroviral agents for HIV PEP should be available for timely administration.

Health care workers should be told to report occupational exposures immediately after they occur, particularly because HBIG, hepatitis B vaccine, and HIV PEP are most likely to be effective if administered as soon after the exposure as possible.

14. How can occupational exposures be prevented?

Approximately 600,000–800,000 needlestick injuries occur in the United States annually. Health care workers should assume that blood and other body fluids from all patients are potentially infectious. They should follow infection control precautions at all times. These precautions include the routine use of barriers when contact with blood or body fluids is anticipated, washing hands and other skin surfaces immediately after contact with blood or body fluids, and the careful handling and disposing of sharp instruments during and after use. Safety devices also have been developed to help prevent needle-stick injuries. If used properly, these types of devices may reduce the occupational HIV exposure risk.

OSHA published the *Occupational Exposure to Bloodborne Pathogens Standard* in 1991 because of a significant health risk associated with exposure to viruses and other microorganisms that cause bloodborne diseases. Many medical devices have been developed to reduce the risk of needlesticks and sharps injuries. Despite these advances in technology, needlesticks and other sharps injuries continue to be of concern because of their high frequency and the severity of the health effects.[10]

In response to both the continued concern about such exposures and the technologic developments that can increase employee protection, Congress passed the Needlestick Safety and Prevention Act in January, 2001. This act directs OSHA to revise the bloodborne pathogens standard and establish in greater detail requirements that employers identify and make use of effective and safer medical devices. The revision, which became effective in April, 2001, added new requirements for employers, including additions to the exposure control plan, employee input, documentation of employee input, and keeping a sharps injury log. The complete list of regulations can be found at www.osha.gov/needlesticks/needlefact.html.

15. What are the recommendations for exposures that do not occur at work?

In 1992 the CDC published guidelines entitled *Management of Possible Sexual, Injecting-Drug-Use, or Other Non-occupational Exposure to HIV, Including Considerations Related to Antiretroviral Therapy.* The United States Public Health Service (USPHS) has concluded that no data address the effectiveness of antiretroviral therapy in preventing HIV transmission after non-occupational exposures. USPHS believes that this lack of data makes definitive recommendations impossible. Because the therapy remains unproven and poses significant risks, physicians should consider its use only in extreme circumstances when the probability of HIV infection is high. The therapy can be initiated promptly when adherence to the regimen is likely.

After noting several instances of HIV transmission after rape, New York State determined that victims and practitioners would benefit from standardized guidelines that address HIV prophylaxis after sexual assault. In June, 1998 the New York State Department of Health AIDS Institute published *HIV Prophylaxis Following Sexual Assault: Guidelines for Adults and Adolescents.*[5]

Survivors of sexual assault should be considered candidates for HIV PEP when significant exposure may have occurred, as defined by direct contact of the vagina, anus, or mouth with the semen or blood of the perpetrator, with or without physical injury, tissue damage, or presence of blood at the site of the assault. PEP should be offered as soon as possible after exposure, ideally within 1 hour; it should not be offered 36 hours or more after the exposure.[5] These guidelines are available at www.hivguidelines.org.

16. How does PEP for sexual assault differ from PEP for occupational exposure?

Unique challenges are associated with PEP after sexual assault:
- **Perpetrator.** In occupational exposure, the HIV status of the source patient is considered. In sexual assault. the recommendation for PEP is based on the nature of the exposure and the survivor's ability to complete the regimen.
- **HIV testing.** Most sexual assault survivors are seen in the emergency department (ED). With occupational exposure, employee health and infection control practitioners are available to assist the worker. In a sexual assault, the HIV testing and pretest counseling need to be done in the ED.
- **Cost.** The cost of PEP is about $800 for a two-drug regimen and $1200 for a three-drug regimen. In occupational exposure, the employer is responsible for payment. In sexual assaults, the survivor is responsible for payment.
- **Side effects.** The possibility of side effects from PEP increases substantially with the addition of emergency contraception and antibiotics prescribed for prophylaxis of sexually transmitted diseases.

• **Team work.** To create a seamless system for PEP after sexual assault, the following resources must be included in creating and implementing the plan: law enforcement agencies, emergency responders, rape crisis volunteers, emergency department staff, social workers, pharmacists, and community physicians.

17. How is PEP for sexual assault similar to PEP for occupational exposure?

When it is determined the sexual assault survivor meets the criteria for and accepts PEP, the protocol is the same as for occupational exposure. Counseling, lab tests, and follow-up remain the same.

18. What is a rapid source of current information about PEP?

The recommendations about PEP after occupational exposure or sexual assault are continually being updated. For the latest information check www.cdc/gov. PEP after occupational exposure and sexual assault is crucial for prevention of HIV transmission. Implementing these guidelines is not without challenges. Knowing and planning for these common challenges increase the chances that the guidelines will be implemented in a timely manner, patients will continue PEP without interruption, and therapy will be completed. Employers need to create clear and concise policies and procedures, educate staff about their implementation, and make every effort to prevent occupational exposures.

BIBLIOGRAPHY

1. Centers for Disease Control and Prevention: Case-control study of HIV seroconversion in health-care workers after percutaneous exposure to HIV-infected blood—France, United Kingdom, and United States, January 1988–August 1994. MMWR 44 (RR50): 929–933, 1995.
2. Centers for Disease Control and Prevention: Management of possible sexual, injecting-drug-use, or other nonoccupational exposure to HIV, including considerations related to antiretroviral therapy. Public Health Service Statement. MMWR, 47(RR17), 1–14, 1998.
3. Centers for Disease Control and Prevention: Updated U.S. Public Health Service guidelines for the management of occupational exposures to HBV, HCV and HIV and recommendations for postexposure prophylaxis. MMWR 50 (RR11):1–52, 2001.
4. Department of Health and Human Services: Exposure to Blood: What Health-Care Workers Need to Know [brochure]. Washington, DC, Department of Health and Human Services.
5. New York State AIDS Institute" HIV Prophylaxis following Sexual Assault: Guidelines for Adults and Adolescent [publication 9315]. Albany, NY, New York State AIDS Institute, 1998.
6. New York State AIDS Institute: HIV Prophylaxis following Occupational Exposure: Guidelines for Adults and Adolescents [publication 9316]. Albany, NY, New York State AIDS Institute, 2001
7. Occupational Safety and Health Administration: Revision to OSHA's Bloodborne Pathogens Standard, Technical Background and Summary. Available at www.osha.gov/needlesticks/needlefact.html. 2001.
8. Proia L, Kessler H: Rationale and recommendations for HIV postexposure prophylaxis. Infect Med 18 (9): 428–438, 2001.
9. Sperling RS, et al: Pediatric AIDS clinical trials group protocol 076 study group. Maternal viral load, zidovudine treatment and the risk of transmission of human immunodeficiency virus from mother to infant. N Engl J Med 335 (22):1621–1629, 1996.
10. Wang SA, et al: Experience of healthcare workers taking postexposure prophylaxis after occupational exposures: Findings of the HIV postexposure prophylaxis registry infection control. Hosp Epidemiol 21:780, 2000.

9. ETHICAL AND LEGAL ISSUES

Elizabeth Anne Mahoney, RN, MS, EdD, ACRN

Ethical and legal issues that are relevant for all nursing practice are related despite their differences. *Ethics* refers to the moral or good of human conduct in a specific situation. *Legal* refers to statutes, laws, and regulations, such as nurse practice acts. Sometimes ethical and legal issues may be similar; at other times, they may be in opposition. Maintaining client confidentiality is required by the national and international codes for nurses[1,6] and the American Nurses Association's (ANA) standards of nursing practice[2] as well as by federal and state laws, including some professional practice acts.[3] The ANA's position statement and many nurses' moral beliefs are in opposition to patient-assisted suicide (PAS), yet PAS is legal in Oregon and the Netherlands.

1. What are the two major theories related to ethics?

Utilitarianism (teleology) focuses on the short- and long-term outcomes of an action in light of the greatest good for the greatest number. Triage and public health policy are based on this theory that the end justifies the means. People may be means rather than ends; for example, when one of the groups in an antiretroviral drug-dose research study receives a placebo medication.

In contrast, **deontology** focuses on duty and the consistent application of principles in all situations. Deontologists ensure autonomy in decision making for all competent persons, regardless of the anticipated outcome. The person is the end in this theory.[6]

2. How are the major principles of ethics relevant to persons with HIV/AIDS?

Major ethical principles include autonomy, paternalism/parentalism, confidentiality, beneficence/nonmaleficence, veracity, sanctity of life/duty to care, and justice. Some principles have legal as well as ethical aspects.

3. Describe autonomy.

Autonomy is the right of each person who is capable of making informed choices to make decisions related to his or her life and treatment. Autonomy necessitates that the person is informed of available options, all positive and/or negative consequences, and the possible results of declining treatment (informed refusal). Information should not be withheld based on the client's age, gender, sexual orientation/preference, race, or ethnicity. Client autonomy places the responsibility for communicating clear information on the provider and the responsibility for decision making on the client.

Client education has a major effect on autonomy. For example, the client with HIV/AIDS must be informed of the drugs used in treatment, the number of pills/doses to be taken during the day, timing of medications, possible side effects, interactions with other medications that the person is taking, and supports available before committing to a therapeutic regimen.

4. Define paternalism and parentalism. How do they relate to autonomy?

Paternalism embraces the belief that the provider knows best, much as in a parent-child relationship. Indeed, the term *parentalism* is now recommended to avoid the gender bias of paternalism.[6] The provider is the decision maker and may be selective in the information shared with the client; the provider may decide that limited information is "all the person needs to know or can understand." In this situation the provider may not want to or may not take the time to translate the information so that the client can understand. Paternalism/parentalism can be justified only if the person is unable to make decisions, if no harm will occur to the client by the paternalistic act, or if telling a client would cause serious harm (e. g., a client would commit suicide if told that he or she had HIV/AIDS).

Autonomy and paternalism/parentalism are at opposite ends of the decision-making contin-uum. Autonomy empowers the client, paternalism places the client in a subservient position. In contrast to the educational approach of autonomy (see question 2), the paternalistic/parentalistic approach provides information about the medication schedule that the provider has prepared, em-phasizing the need to be compliant. Another example is withholding a prognosis because the client "could not understand" all of the ramifications.

5. Describe confidentiality. Why is it a particular concern for people with HIV/AIDS?

Confidentiality refers to the responsibility of the health care provider to respect the client's privacy and to share only with persons who have a right to know only the information that they need to know. Maintaining confidentiality provides a foundation for building trust and a positive client-provider relationship. In this aspect, confidentiality is similar for all clients, regardless of the diagnosis. Health care providers should not discuss client information in areas where others, lay or agency persons, can hear (e.g., nurses' stations, hallways, elevators, cafeterias, restaurants, or any public setting or with family members or friends without the client's permission).

Maintaining the client's confidence is particularly important for people with HIV/AIDS be-cause of specific issues, including stigma and fear of loss of work and health benefits. Therefore, some of the first questions asked of the client with HIV/AIDS include the following: Who knows your diagnosis? Who can be told medical information? Can messages be left with others or on answering machines? Chapters related to vulnerable populations, particularly infants, children, adolescents, women, and people with HIV behind bars, discuss ways that confidentiality may be breached based on organizational policy.

Frequently the nurse is in a dilemma to know how and with whom to communicate about the client's status. Clearly addressing these questions during the initial visit and when changes occur can prevent potential problems. Nurses may experience ethical dilemmas when a client does not wish to notify sexual contacts of his or her HIV/AIDS status for fear of abandonment or reprisal, yet the contact has a right to know of his or her risk. The nurse can discuss with the client issues related to sharing information about the diagnosis with those who need to know and teach harm-reducing behaviors to decrease risk of transmission.

6. Summarize beneficence and nonmaleficence.

Beneficence and nonmaleficence are two sides of the same issue. Beneficence refers to "doing good," whereas nonmaleficence refers to "avoiding harm."

Beneficence is a guiding principle when a person who has been exposed to HIV through a needlestick injury is immediately informed of the risk, told of the postexposure protocol, and provided access to the appropriate treatment and follow-up. Another example relates to the in-creasing incidence of sexually transmitted diseases (STDs) among adolescents. Nurses in the U.S. have stated that health care providers have an ethical responsibility to provide comprehen-sive, prevention-focused education about STDs and HIV to this population.[4] In England and Wales, the Education Act of 1996 mandates that sex education in schools must include teaching about STDs and HIV as well as sex and marriage.[11]

Nonmaleficence is exhibited by the health care provider who refuses to help a person with HIV/AIDS commit suicide. Of course, some persons argue that such action is paternalism and a violation of the client's autonomy; hence the term *ethical dilemma* or *conflict in values*. Complying with a client's request for assisted suicide also raises legal issues in most of the United States (Oregon is an exception) and many other countries (the Netherlands is an excep-tion). Nonmaleficence also is a key principle in clinical trials and other research. Subjects should not be at risk for harm in any study group.[5] Withholding proven treatment (e.g., information, drugs) for the sake of research is unethical. The Tuskegee syphilis study is a classic example of maleficence.

Beneficence and nonmaleficence are related to the New York State law that requires the availability of counseling resources when HIV test results (positive or negative) are disclosed to a client.[8]

7. Describe veracity.

Veracity or truth-telling means that health care providers are honest in communication with their clients and each other. Some may argue that not telling the truth is justified if the truth would have a negative effect on the client (similar to a paternalistic/parentalistic attitude). Veracity means informing the client that he or she has HIV and explaining the options and their consequences. Truth-telling is closely allied to autonomy and informed consent/refusal. Thus, the person must have sufficient, accurate information on which to base a decision.

8. What are the implications of the sanctity of human life and duty to care?

The sanctity of human life and duty to care are integral principles for all health care professions, closely related to beneficence. Sanctity of life refers to the belief in the inherent worth of each individual.[12] Duty to care means that all providers have the responsibility to care for each person presented for treatment, regardless of demographic variables and diagnosis. These principles were severely tested in the early years of the epidemic in the United States when many health care workers refused to participate in the care of persons with HIV/AIDS, including bringing and removing food trays, providing personal care, or touching the person without gloves.

Nonmaleficence may supersede duty to care in some situations. A nurse may ethically refuse to care for an HIV/AIDS client because of religious beliefs or if the risk of harm is greater than the client's benefit from the care.[10]

Sanctity of life and duty to care mean that nurses treat all clients with dignity and respect, provide timely care, provide prompt medication for pain so that the client does not seek an end to life as a means of ending pain, and, in the U.S., implement the ANA Code of Ethics[1] and Standards of Clinical Nursing Practice.[2]

9. Discuss justice.

Justice is the principle of fairness in the distribution of resources, especially scarce assets.[6,12] Resources include time, money, effort, and people. Research and other funding have promoted pharmaceutical development, geno- and phenotyping, testing, and other monitoring and treatment modalities for people with HIV/AIDS. Justice necessitates that the resources and personnel knowledgeable about HIV/AIDS be available to treat infected people and work to prevent further spread of the disease. Others argue that sufficient resources are being expended and that other chronic conditions must receive equal funding. Justice is compatible with a deontologic perspective.

10. What are some of the most common legal issues for persons with HIV/AIDS?

Some of the most common legal issues for people with HIV/AIDS include disclosure with the related aspects of confidentiality and privacy, informed consent, discrimination, access to care, and end-of-life decisions.

11. What are the issues related to disclosure, confidentiality, and privacy?

Disclosure is an encompassing term that refers to revealing or exposing information about a person without permission. The disclosure frequently is written or verbal but may include using photographs or names for unsanctioned advertising or media release. Discussing a man's progress in HIV treatment with new clients, without his permission, is an example of disclosure. Before 1996, New York State mandated testing of all newborns for statistical purposes but did not share the results with parents.[12] Now names are attached to the results.[8] Although most states provide for some disclosure of HIV/AID-related information (e.g., for state databases, criminal charges), nurses should be informed about the legal aspects of disclosure in their specific state(s). Disclosure is a frequent dilemma for nurses,[7] who may experience a conflict between the client's and partner's right to know the client's HIV/AIDS status.

Many people, including health care personnel, argue that knowing the HIV/AIDS status of clients would allow them to take extra safety measures to protect themselves from risk. The Occupational Safety and Health Administration (OSHA) standard 29 CFR 1910.1030 mandates employers' and employees' use of universal precautions as a means of limiting contact with infected blood and body fluids. Fines can be assessed for failure to comply with the standard.[9] Adherence to the standard negates the need to know a diagnosis and the risk of fine. Indeed, people are more at risk from those who have not yet been diagnosed with an infectious disease. Universal precautions is a harm-reduction measure for all situations.

Confidentiality is a legal as well as an ethical issue. Its definition in both cases means that health care providers must respect the client's privacy and share with persons who have a right to know only the information that they need to know. Discussing the client's status with family members, significant others, other staff who are not involved in the client's care, or people who inquire about the client is illegal and a breach of the client-provider privilege.

Privacy refers to the right of the person to control what, where, and when personal information is shared.[6] The U.S. Privacy Act requires the written request or permission of the client before any of his or her records in the federal system can be disclosed.[3]

12. How does informed consent apply to persons with HIV/AIDS?

Informed consent refers to the client's voluntary agreement to a plan based on clear, understandable information. The opposite, informed refusal, is the client's voluntary decision not to participate in a plan based on clear, understandable information about the consequences of such a choice. Understandable information is essential for either choice.

Informed consent is similar for persons with and without HIV/AIDS. In the U.S., failure to officially classify HIV/AIDS as a communicable disease with mandatory reporting and informing contacts of their risk has led to much controversy as well as ethical and legal issues. Some of the key decisions for people with HIV/AIDS include testing to determine HIV/AIDS status, adhering to a medication regimen, telling a partner or family member of the diagnosis, and participating in research studies. In most states, client consent is needed for HIV/AIDS testing. However, exceptions include autopsies, protection of caregivers, body tissue/fluid donations, criteria for some jobs, anonymous research,[10] and (in New York) felons who are guilty of forcing sexual intercourse on an unwilling recipient.[8]

Informing a spouse and/or partner about a client's HIV/AIDS status is a controversial legal and ethical issue. Conflict exists between the client's right to confidentiality and informed consent and the spouse or partner's right to know his or her risk.

Most states do not mandate that health care providers notify sexual contacts of their risk.[10] In some states and countries (such as Uganda),[13] health care providers, including nurses, legally cannot reveal the client's HIV/AIDS status without consent, regardless of the risk to others. However, many states allow exceptions to the rule of disclosing the client's HIV/AIDS status without permission. Texas indicates with whom positive results can be shared.[10] New York allows physicians to reveal a client's HIV/AIDS status to contacts who are in jeopardy of acquiring HIV/AIDS from a client who will not disclose his or her status voluntarily.[8]

Autonomy and respect for the rights of others are key ethical principles in informed consent. As a result, the nurse may explore with the client the conflict of rights and look for ways to resolve the situation without rejecting the client for his or her desire not to tell.

13. Why is discrimination an issue for clients with HIV/AIDS?

Discrimination is the "unfair treatment or denial of privileges to persons because of their sex, age, race, nationality, or religion"[10] (p. 536). Chronic health conditions have been added to the list by the Americans with Disabilities Act (ADA) of 1990. This act prohibits discrimination against persons with disabilities, including HIV/AIDS, by employers who have 15 or more employees.[3,10] Lack of knowledge, fear, and anger at persons whose sexual or drug-use lifestyles place them at risk have led to discrimination among people with HIV/AIDS. Infected persons may be at additional risk for discrimination because of their sex, sexual orientation, or race.

Results of discrimination include loss or denial of jobs; loss or denial of health benefits or health care coverage; isolation from family, friends, and communities; loss of or lack of access to housing; and marginalization. Families of persons with HIV/AIDS also suffer discrimination and isolation. Fear of discrimination is a major reason why clients do not want to disclose their positive HIV/AIDS status.

14. Why is access to care an issue?

Access to care is an issue for many people. Outcomes of discrimination and the physical, emotional, and mental stresses associated with HIV/AIDS compound the situation. A person without a job and income has less or no health benefits or money to pay for care, medications, and normal life expenses and can experience decreased self-concept. Even people with current employment and health insurance have no guarantees that either will continue. The client fears loss of these resources. Debilitation, lack of convenient transportation, and distance also interfere with access. Availability of qualified health care personnel to treat HIV/AIDS and its sequelae is another major impediment to receiving appropriate care.

Clients must exhaust most of their savings to qualify for Medicaid benefits. Monies available to states through Title XXVI of the Public Health Service Act are contingent on states meeting certain criteria, including legal mandates for partner notification (for Ryan White funds).[12] Helping clients access care involves a multidisciplinary effort, patience, and perseverance.

15. What are some of the end-of-life issues for clients with HIV/AIDS?

End-of-life issues are similar for persons with and without HIV/AIDS. Exceptions include issues such as who is the recipient of any benefits, who holds power of attorney or is the defined health care proxy, and who implements the living will. Frequently this person may not be a family member, and conflicts with relatives may arise in the implementation of the client's wishes. Consulting with an attorney to make a will and safeguard the client's intents is essential. Providing for care and guardianship of children is crucial. Some states allow a standby guardian who may take care of children when the parent is hospitalized and return custody when the parent is able to resume this responsibility. Exploring options and preplanning are critical to ensure that the client's intents are realized.

Ethical and legal issues provide challenges for clients with HIV/AIDS, spouses and partners, relatives, nurses, and other health care providers. Knowledge, mutual respect, and collaboration can help convert challenges into opportunities for successful outcomes.

BIBLIOGRAPHY

1. American Nurses Association: Code of Ethics for Nurses with Interpretive Statements. Washington, DC, American Nurses Association, 2002.
2. American Nurses Association: Standards of Clinical Nursing Practice, 2nd ed. Washington, DC, American Nurses Association, 1998.
3. Brent NJ: Nurses and the Law, 2nd ed. Philadelphia, W.B. Saunders, 2001.
4. Browne EJ, Simpson EM: Comprehensive STD/HIV prevention education targeting US adolescents: Review of an ethical dilemma and proposed ethical framework. Nurs Ethics 7(4):339–349, 2000.
5. Bryan C: AIDS expert challenges ethical stance on drug trials. Br Med J 323:531, 2001.
6. Burkhardt MA, Nathaniel AK: Ethics and Issues in Contemporary Nursing. Albany, NY, Delmar, 1998.
7. Garcia JG, Forrester LE, Jacob AV: Ethical dilemma resolution in HIV/AIDS counseling: Why an integrative model? Int J Rehabil Health 4(3):167–181, 1998.
8. Gold BA: New York Health Law, 2nd ed. Albany, NY, Fort Orange Press, 1997.
9. Nielsen RP: OSHA Regulations and Guidelines: A Guide for Health Care Providers. Albany, NY, Delmar, 2000.
10. O'Keefe ME: Nursing Practice and the Law. Philadelphia, F.A. Davis, 2001.
11. Sex Education Legislation for Schools in England and Wales. Available at http:// www.avert.org/legislation.htm. Accessed May 30, 2002.
12. Ungvarski PJ, Flaskerud JH (eds): HIV/AIDS: A Guide to Primary Care Management, 4th ed. Philadelphia, W.B., Saunders, 1999.
13. Vogel G: Study of HIV transmission sparks ethics debate. N Engl J Med 288:22–23, 2000.

10. HIV/AIDS AND SPIRITUALITY

Mary Anne Brown, RN, BSN, MA

Whether we are physically unhealthy, emotionally broken, or spiritually barren, we experience a condition of incompleteness that is neither wholesome nor healthy. Serious illness often triggers a spiritual crisis. The person with HIV/AIDS is facing physical and emotional challenges that are clearly evident and generally are well addressed in the health care providers' plan of care. Sadly, the spiritual dimension of a client's health is usually left to chance or disregarded as falling into the realm of the ordained clergy. The nursing profession, however, is no stranger to the concept of caring for the whole person. Nursing maintains a philosophy, fostered by Florence Nightingale, that includes the care of the physical, emotional, and spiritual needs of the whole person. Although nursing theory is still not commonly used in all practice settings, research and professional writing have prompted a renewed interest and recognition of the influence of wholeness and health in the continuum of health care. In HIV/AIDS nursing, caring for spiritual needs is a significant component of the well-being of clients. Indeed, attending to spiritual needs is as essential as rendering physical and psychological care.

1. What is the relationship among faith, spirituality, and health?

There are as many understandings of faith as there are people, for no one can characterize faith for another person. In general, however, faith is considered an experience and an awareness of the divine. The divine may be God, a Higher Power, or an eternal force that is holy and untouchable. Spirituality is a life-defining attitude that involves faith in a supernatural being or presence as well as a realization of love and connection with others. It gives meaning to life and provides an understanding of death. It offers a sense of hope and direction throughout life.

Because the body, mind, and spirit are equal components of humans, faith and spirituality have great influence on health and wellness. Wholeness, of course, includes the physical, mental, and spiritual. Studies support the value of spiritual health and its role in fostering healthier outcomes for people with serious illnesses. Ellison concluded that religion enhances well-being through social and spiritual relationships and by providing meaning in life and "existential certainty."[5] Social, religious, and existential well-being has been positively linked to a well population.[8,9] Indeed, spirituality is a time-honored resource that helps people with chronic illnesses (including HIV/AIDS) to cope with the physiologic and psychological difficulties of disease.

2. What are the key components of spiritual care?

Spiritual care encompasses a number of activities that are within the realm of the nursing process:
- Assessment of spiritual needs
- Planning nursing management of the nursing diagnosis of spiritual distress[1]
- Implementation of nursing intervention
- Evaluation of spiritual care outcomes

Assessment of spiritual needs often begins during the initial encounter with the client and continues throughout the client's illness.

3. Define spiritual distress.

Spiritual distress is a state of disruption in a belief or value system that provides strength, hope, and meaning to life and that transcends individual biologic and psychosocial nature.

4. What key assessment findings indicate spiritual distress?
- The client questions the meaning of life and death or a belief system.
- The client expresses concern about his or her relationship with God.

• The client addresses anger toward staff, family, God, or religious figures.
• The client demonstrates behavior and/or mood changes.
• The client complains of sleep disturbances or nightmares.
• The client requests spiritual assistance.

The stigma of the disease intensifies the spiritual concerns of the HIV/AIDS client. Often the prejudice and rejection displayed by family and society toward the client's homosexual or drug-using lifestyle can trigger a spiritual crisis. People with HIV/AIDS have not yet achieved the level of family and social support commonly experienced by other chronically or terminally ill clients, particularly during the difficult periods of drug therapy, pain management, and the dying experience. Recognizing the high potential for social isolation and rejection is particularly essential during the spiritual assessment of the client infected with HIV/AIDS.

5. How can the nurse plan and implement care for a client in spiritual distress?

Once the nursing diagnosis of spiritual distress is made, the nurse can begin a plan of care. Its implementation focuses on the following elements:
• Nonjudgmental communication
• Establishing with the client a plan of achievable goals
• Providing spiritual support
• Engaging other spiritual resources.

6. How does the nurse know that the nursing interventions were effective?

Outcome criteria of nursing interventions used to diminish spiritual distress are measured by the client's response. Clearly, if the findings in the spiritual assessment are lessened (the client is more restful, less agitated, and more hopeful), the nursing care plan has been effective.

7. What barriers to providing spiritual care are commonly encountered in nursing practice? How do they particularly affect patients with HIV/AIDS?

Nurses can overlook the spiritual dimension in the care of a client for a number of reasons: perceived lack of time, insufficient knowledge to apply any spiritual nursing intervention, misperception that spirituality is a socially inappropriate topic to discuss in a professional setting, and personal attitudes toward their own and others' spiritual concerns.

Another barrier to incorporating the spiritual dimension into the plan of care may be the nurse's anxiety and reluctance. Before working with the homosexual and drug-using population, the nursing professional must first resolve any personal issues of conflict that may interfere with professional care of clients with HIV/AIDS. A nonjudgmental, accepting attitude facilitates the general well-being of the client.

8. What if the client claims no religion?

Spiritual assessment is not complete at the end of the initial examination. Often if an admission assessment form asks for the client's religion and the client answers "none," no additional exploration of spiritual needs occurs. However, belonging to a particular faith tradition is not the sole indicator of spirituality, and the assessment of spiritual needs must continue throughout the plan of care.

9. Is the spiritual care of clients truly within the realm of nursing practice?

As professionals who are patient-centered and wholistic in practice, nurses can quite naturally attend to the spiritual needs of a client. Nurses spend considerable time with clients and are able to establish the trust and understanding that become the foundation for sharing on a deeper level. Health is indeed a spiritual issue. Nursing care and service are not divergent but are interdependent and mutually strengthening in the delivery of health care. The nursing profession by its history has embraced wholeness rather than cure as a philosophy, and the spiritual component is key to wholeness. In Christian faiths, Jesus did not ask the man at Bethesda if he wanted a cure or to be rid of his ailment. He asked instead, "Do you want to be made well?" In turn, nursing encourages an attitude of wellness (wholeness) to become sound of body, mind, and spirit, unbroken and restored so that those for whom we care will be strong and complete to face what life brings. People who face the challenges of terminal illness, in particular HIV/AIDS, generally recognize that cure may be unlikely, but treatment measures, symptom management, and an overall sensible approach provide comfort and a sense of well-being.

Nurses are not alone in attending to spiritual health. Providing spiritual care to clients is a shared role and, indeed, there are times when other members of the health team (e.g., chaplain, pastoral care counselor, clergy) are asked to serve the client who is in spiritual crisis.

10. How is the psychosocial dimension distinct from the spiritual dimension of a client assessment and plan of care?

Although spiritual distress is often revealed through emotions, emotional support alone does not help the client whose difficulty is principally spiritual. Although both the psychosocial and the spiritual focus on the person's ability to cope with the emotional aspects of illness and its crises, the distinction has everything to do with relationships.

The psychosocial assessment examines the client's relationship with family, friends, and community. The psychosocial plan of care focuses on assisting the client to cope more effectively with psychological and social variables during stressful times. Although spiritual dimensions are often identified during the initial psychosocial assessment, the spiritual assessment and plan of care take place within the context of the client's belief system and relationship to self and God (e.g., Higher Power, eternal force). Spiritual interventions incorporate the psychosocial nursing skills of listening, empathy, and openness and foster the client's comfort through the expression of personal spiritual and religious values, beliefs, and practices.

11. Distinguish among faith, spirituality, and religion.

Simply stated, **faith** is the experience of the divine. **Spirituality** is the influence of this faith experience on the person's life and is illustrated through attitudes, values, and health. **Religion** is the organized creed of the tradition, held by members within the circle of the particular faith tradition. The nursing professional who explores his or her own beliefs and sense of the spiritual is better prepared to intervene with clients experiencing spiritual distress.

12. What are some religious beliefs that may affect nursing care?

In caring for clients, the nursing professional must convey nonjudgmental acceptance of a broad variety of spiritual and cultural beliefs and customs. Many of the faith traditions hold beliefs about birth and death, diet and food practices, medical care, and clinical decision-making that the attentive nurse will respect while planning and providing care. It is important to know whether a certain faith tradition requires or opposes infant baptism, what rituals are expected at death, the fasting and food restrictions that are followed, and whether medical therapy is restricted in certain circumstances. Examples of traditions with specific beliefs and practices are listed below. A more comprehensive listing is available from Public Health and Community Health Nurse's Consultant.[12]

Traditions with Beliefs and Practices That Affect Nursing Care

TRADITION	BELIEFS ABOUT BIRTH-DEATH	FOOD PRACTICES	MEDICAL CARE
Adventist	✓	✓	✓
Baptist	✓	✓	✓
Black Muslim	✓	✓	✓
Buddhist	✓		✓
Christian Science	✓		✓
Mormon	✓	✓	✓
Eastern Orthodox	✓	✓	

Table continued on following page

Traditions with Beliefs and Practices That Affect Nursing Care (Continued)

TRADITION	BELIEFS ABOUT BIRTH-DEATH	FOOD PRACTICES	MEDICAL CARE
Episcopal	✓	✓	
Quakers			
Greek Orthodox	✓	✓	✓
Hindu	✓	✓	
Islam	✓	✓	✓
Jehovah's Witnesses		✓	✓
Judaism	✓	✓	✓
Lutheran	✓		
Presbyterian	✓		
Roman Catholic	✓	✓	✓
Russian Orthodox	✓	✓	✓

13. How do clients express spiritual needs and manifest spiritual distress?

Spiritual needs emerge when a client lacks any factor needed to maintain a sense of self, an awareness of the divine, or an experience of love. The client with HIV/AIDS may have already encountered religious alienation because of lifestyle. This abandonment causes an even greater need for spiritual comfort, yet the client, confused and angered by past treatment received from members and leaders of a faith community, has difficulty in trusting others with sensitive news about his or her HIV status. When life loses meaning or when hope for the future is absent, a client may express doubt, fear, and even despair. The nurse assesses these needs by observing and listening in an atmosphere of trust. A client may display anger toward God or religious representatives. He or she may reveal a fear of dying or become withdrawn and unable to concentrate during conversations. A client may be extremely apprehensive or deny any emotions or worries. Indicators of spiritual distress may be subtle or quite evident. By using listening, observation, and assessment skills, the alert nursing professional will be able to meet many of these needs and will collaborate with other spiritual care team members whenever appropriate.

14. How does a nursing professional conduct a spiritual assessment?

Assessment of a client's spirituality can be organized into six components:

- **Conduct and/or appearance** (religious articles and reading evident in client's environment; engagement in rituals to the exclusion of interaction with others; frequent reference to religious topics while talking with others; withdrawal; lethargy; suicidal ideation; increase in alcohol intake)
- **Emotions** (high level of anxiety; denial of emotions or worries; anger with God; blaming God for the suffering; feeling hopeless or helpless)
- **Concepts, beliefs, and understanding** (feeling overwhelmed with situation/life and thinking nothing can help; concluding that he or she has committed unforgivable sins; narcissism; professing to hear voices of religious figures)
- **Relationships and contacts** (feelings of detachment from others; withdrawal from those with dissimilar beliefs; disassociation from family and friends of the same tradition)
- **Physical signs/symptoms** (discomforts; sleeping/eating difficulties)
- **Relevant history** (involvement in faith community/organized tradition; other tragic medical events)

15. What are the essentials of designing a spiritual needs protocol to guide nursing and other health care professionals in providing clients with spiritual support and comfort?

The spiritual needs protocol outlined below is a model policy that may be adapted for use by nursing staff working in a variety of settings throughout the continuum of health care.

Spiritual Needs Protocol

Policy

Assessing and providing for spiritual needs is commonly completed during the initial assessment of a client and at other appropriate times during client encounters.

Purpose

The spiritual dimension is an integral part of a person and, although it is not scientifically validated, it is critical to the wholeness of the person. Spiritual distress may result from illness or injury, regardless of whether a client affiliates with an organized faith tradition

Procedure:	Spiritual needs assessment
Equipment:	Spiritual needs assessment guide
Preparation:	Review spiritual assessment skills.
	Provide a private environment.
	Convey an attitude of trust and confidentiality.
Steps:	1. Observe client's conduct, appearance, and environment.
	2. Determine level of client's emotional state.
	3. Listen for client's concepts, beliefs, and perceptions of life in the context of this illness/injury.
	4. Consider client's relationships and contacts and observe client's interaction within these relationships.
	5. Observe physical signs/symptoms.
	6. Obtain any other relevant history.
	7. Prepare an appropriate plan of nursing intervention that includes collaboration with a chaplain, clergy, and others who will assist in the effective care of client's spiritual needs.

Client and family teaching

Instruct client and family about how to blend religious practices into the health plan of care (e.g., nutrition and dietary practices). Support religious customs and practices, and encourage family/friends to do so. On discharge, refer to a suitable clergy representative, if indicated and agreeable to client.

Documentation

Record client's conclusion in terms of the illness/injury, strife within network of family/friends. Record client's reaction to clergy visit.

---

16. What is the relevance of spirituality to the plan of care for HIV clients?

Experience and research have underscored that, when confronted with the life-threatening illness of HIV/AIDS, clients encounter a myriad of challenges that strike at the heart of their spirituality. They must face the issues of a terminal disease. Also, because of the bias and fear that accompanies the disease, family, friends, and religious communities often stigmatize them. Clients also may view HIV/AIDS as a punishment for a lifestyle that is inconsistent with a religious or spiritual tradition or as abandonment by a Supreme Being. With such a burden of loss, accompanied by social and spiritual isolation, people with HIV/AIDS have an acute need for the management of spiritual distress to be included in their plan of care.

17. With so many pressing clinical concerns related to the HIV/AIDS disease process, why would a nursing professional address spirituality in a client's plan of care?

The wholistic philosophy of attending the needs of the body, mind, and spirit is fundamental to the effective nursing care of the client with HIV/AIDS. As John Steinbeck wrote, "A sad soul can kill you quicker, far quicker than a germ."[11] Research supports this notion. Increasing evidence documents that by meeting and supporting spiritual and psychosocial needs within the overall plan of care, the client with HIV/AIDS is more prepared to cope with the challenges of a demanding disease.[2,10] Through the interventions offered to relieve spiritual distress, the nurse helps the client to realize a sense of purpose, to grieve the physical and emotional losses, and to address the many issues confronted during the stages of HIV/AIDS. Indeed, spirituality plays a central role in the clinical management of the client with HIV/AIDS.

18. How can nursing professionals become more effective in addressing the spiritual care needs of HIV clients?

Before one can become more confident in spiritual assessment and intervention, the nursing professional must begin with a spiritual self-assessment. How one defines faith, experiences God, fosters a spiritual nature, and relates to religious custom will influence the spiritual interventions with clients. A number of tools are available (Reed's Spiritual Perspective Scale,[2,10] Elkins' Spiritual Orientation Inventory[3,4]) that can measure spiritual perspective and provide a basis for furthering spirituality and ability to meet the spiritual needs of others. The nurse must personally resolve issues of faith, prayer, ritual, life choices, and high-risk behavior in a client and religious beliefs and practices that conflict with his or her own moral principles in order to address spiritual needs fittingly. The nursing professional who is present, attentive, and understanding while caring for the client with HIV/AIDS provides the more favorable environment for the client's spiritual well-being.

19. What interventions are likely be effective in a plan of care that addresses spiritual needs commonly identified in HIV disease (e.g., terminal illness, end-of-life issues, religious/family disenfranchisement, community isolation)?

Spiritual care is the unscientific realm of care that cannot be ignored if healing of the whole person is to occur. The plan of spiritual care for the client with HIV/AIDS uses the nursing process in response to special issues of the disease and its impact on the spirituality of the client:

Assessment
• Identify spiritual needs of the client.
• Be alert and sensitive to disenfranchisement by family and faith community.
• Maintain an accepting and caring manner.
• Observe client's environment (for religious items, Bible), cultural orientation, and social interactions.
• Gauge client's mood and emotion.
• Learn about client's spiritual perceptions.

Planning
• Simply be with the client to listen to his or her concerns and fear.
• Allow the client to vent anger or frustration.
• Offer to join the client in prayer or reading sacred writings.[6]
• Assist the client in obtaining and using religious articles.
• Involve other resources, including spiritual leaders, if the client agrees.

Intervention
• Implement the plan

Outcome criteria
• Client describes feelings about spiritual values, conflict, issues, and sources of strength and peace.
• Client indicates the calming influence of spiritual intervention.
• Client continues suggested spiritual experiences and practices offered during the intervention.

Evaluation
• The effectiveness of the spiritual care intervention is measured by comparing client outcomes and resulting attitude with outcome criteria. For example, the client is more accepting of diagnosis, communicates hope for the future, and acknowledges issues with religion or religious representatives.

20. Summarize practical recommendations for nursing professionals to apply and resources to use in the spiritual care of the HIV/AIDS population.

The basic guidance and resources for nurses providing spiritual care can be summarized in the following pearls:
• **Know thyself.** Explore and crystallize your own personal anxieties and views of HIV/AIDS, sexual mores, drug use, death and dying, and religious differences.

- **Create a caring environment.** Convey an attitude of acceptance and sensitivity and be an attentive listener.
- **Appreciate the stages of the disease.** Spiritual needs differ as the disease advances.
- **Seek further education to enhance counseling skills.** Counseling in the nursing of clients with HIV/AIDS is more intense and requires a deeper focus than that used in general nursing practice.
- **Build strong alliances with other mental health professionals and clergy.** Spiritual care can often be more effective when managed collaboratively.
- **Be appropriate when providing spiritual care.** Appropriate spiritual support is natural, courteous, inoffensive, respectful, and agreeable to the client.

21. What challenges and strengths are encountered by staff in the collaborative management of the spiritual care of clients?

Nurses encounter several challenges in the collaborative management of clients' spiritual care. Sometimes nurses are unprepared or hesitant to include a spiritual component in the plan of care. Perhaps religious representatives impose moral judgement on the client with HIV/AIDS. Because clients may resist meeting with religious representatives, nurses must obtain permission from the client before making a referral to clergy. The result is unmet client needs.

Nursing staff and clergy often complement one another's abilities in meeting spiritual needs, can be mutually supportive, and may benefit the client with HIV/AIDS more completely. Additional strengths include the following:

- Chaplains on staff in health care organizations can provide spiritual counseling and offer the client access to many resources in the community.
- Nurses can rely on chaplains as a support in coping with work stress and health care issues.
- Spiritual representatives from the client's affiliation can be contacted for visits.
- Nurses can develop referral lists of spiritual representatives who provide empathetic support to clients with HIV/AIDS.

The strengths of collaborative management of the spiritual care by clinical and spiritual leaders include a comprehensive, client-centered, well-orchestrated plan of intervention.

22. Can spirituality contribute to the wholeness and wellness of the nurse as well as the client?

Health is a spiritual issue, and, as a spiritual being, the professional nurse can more credibly support an attitude of wholeness by integrating a personal understanding of faith and spirituality. In the teachings of the major faith traditions, each member is called to a greater knowledge and caring of others and self. This message of growth and care is a key principle of health, and how we honor our bodies, minds, and souls will be reflected in the soundness of our individuality. As Miles observed, "Spiritual nurturing contributes to improved life satisfaction and quality of life, improved health, reduced functional disability and lower levels of depression"[7] (p. 24). As people (client and nurse) feel healthier, they feel more open to extending themselves to others who are empty, broken, and in pain.

23. How can nursing professionals cultivate a spiritual dimension in their personal lives?

Caring for the soul or spirit begins with an earnest self-exploration and reflection on the spiritual dimension. Once spiritual needs are identified, the nurse can then begin a plan of self-care that encompasses "soul work," which is the core of true wholeness. The great leaders of faith accept and advocate that true self-love, self-acceptance, and self-regard are the foundation for genuine care of neighbor. The scope of the nursing profession requires that those who serve remain disciplined in practices that will sustain them and keep them whole. Without wholeness, the nurse's love of God, love of self, and love of client will ultimately suffer. Taking care of oneself is not for mere survival, nor is it self-seeking. Being of sound body, mind, and soul is basic to ethical professional nursing. Other essentials for a healthy spirituality include the following:

- Spending time alone and with others praying, meditating, and considering the meaning of life.

- Ongoing spiritual development through reading, discussion, and involvement in small faith communities
- Writing concepts and discoveries of the ways of the spirit in a personal journal
- Serving others in need
- Sharing time regularly with children and older adults
- Walking and spending time in nature
- Attending art exhibits, theatre performances, and musical concerts with spiritual themes

If we tend our bodies with nourishing food, adequate rest, and conscientious exercise, we will respect the gift of the physical. If we care for our minds by allowing, regarding, and accepting our feelings, we will respect the gift of passion. If we magnify our souls through prayer, scripture, and service to others, we will treasure our creator's greatest work.

BIBLIOGRAPHY

1. Carpenito LJ: Handbook of Nursing Diagnosis. Philadelphia, Lippincott, 1999.
2. Castellaw L, Wicks M, Martin J: Spirituality in older women who have osteoarthritis. Spirituality in white older women who have arthritis. Grad Res Nurs [on-line journal], June 1999.
3. Elkins DN: Guidelines for spiritual assessment. Am J Nurs 79:1574–1577, 1979.
4. Elkins DN: Psychotherapy and spirituality: Toward a theory of the soul. J Human Psychol 35(2):78–98, 1995.
5. Ellison C: Spiritual well-being: Conceptualization and measurement. Psychol Theol 11:330–340, 1991.
6. Gorman L, Sultan D, Raines M: Guidelines for use of prayer and religious literature. Davis's Manual of Psychosocial Nursing. Philadelphia, F.A. Davis , 1996.
7. Miles L: Getting started: Parish nursing in a rural community. Christ Nurs 14:24, 1997.
8. Pace J, Stables J: Correlates of spiritual well-being in terminally ill persons with AIDS and terminally ill persons with cancer. J Assoc Nurses AIDS Care 8(6):31–42, 1997.
9. Paloutzian R, Ellison C: Loneliness, spiritual well-being and quality of life. In Peplau L, Perlman D (eds): Loneliness: A Sourcebook of Current Theory, Research, and Therapy. New York, Wiley, 1983.
10. Reed P: Spirituality and well being in terminally ill hospitalized adults. Nurs Rese Health 10:335–344, 1987.
11. Smollin AB: God Knows You're Stressed. Notre Dame, IN, Sorin Books, 2001.
12. Stanhope M, Knollmueller RN: Public Health and Community Health Nurse's Consultant. New York, Mosby, 1997.

II. Compounding the Problem of HIV/AIDS

11. VIRAL HEPATITIS C

Dale S. Ford, RN, MPH, CIC

The hepatitis C virus (HCV) is a ribonucleic acid (RNA) virus of the Flaviviridae family and one of six viruses that together account for the majority of cases of viral hepatitis. HCV infects an estimated 170 million persons worldwide, many of whom are infected with HIV.[6,7,10] Hepatitis C infection, a viral pandemic, is five times as widespread as human immunodeficiency virus type 1 (HIV-1).[7] Since its discovery in 1989, HCV has represented one of the most important causes of chronic liver disease. Blood screening measures have decreased the risk of infection; however, new cases continue to occur, mainly as a result of repeated percutaneous exposures (drug injection) to contaminated blood. Therefore, coinfection with HCV is common (50–90%) among HIV-infected injection drug users.[5,7] Progression from acute to chronic disease occurs in the majority of infected people and has become the major reason for liver transplantation. HCV increases the number of complications in people infected with HIV. Hepatitis C accounts for 8,000–10,000 deaths annually.[1,3,8,9] No vaccine has been developed, and research advances have been impeded by the inability to grow HCV in culture.[7] Treatment modalities, however, have improved.

1. What are the incidence and prevalence of hepatitis C?

Hepatitis C is the most chronic bloodborne pathogen in the United States, affecting approximately 4 million people. Since 1998, the annual incidence of new cases has been estimated at approximately 41,000; hepatitis C accounts for 20% of all viral hepatitis.[6] An estimated 300,000 people are coinfected with HCV and HIV (approximately one-third of the 1 million persons infected with HIV).

Hepatitis C occurs in all populations, with males predominating over females. The highest prevalence rates are in people aged 40–59 years, African-Americans, and/or males.[8] The highest prevalence occurs with those who have repeated percutaneous exposure, including injection drug abusers, hemophiliacs who were treated with clotting factors before discovery of hepatitis C, and recipients of blood transfusions from donors with unknown HCV infection.[1,3]

2. Are transfusions considered a major means of transmission?

At present, transfusions are rarely implicated in the transmission of hepatitis C. After the discovery of hepatitis C, 80% of cases classified as hepatitis non-A and non-B were actually HCV. Since 1985 donors with HIV and non-A, non-B hepatitis have been excluded. In 1990, after the discovery of HCV, screening for antibody to HCV was initiated, and multiantigen tests were implemented in 1992 for further screening of blood donors.[1,3] Coinfection with HIV and HCV was common among persons with hemophilia who received clotting factor concentrates before 1987.[1,3] With screening measures in place, the risk for infection in blood transfusions has been reduced to less than 1 per 100,000 units of blood transfused.[9]

3. What have studies shown to be the predominant modes of transmission?

Studies have shown that injection drug abuse accounts for 60% of HCV transmission and has accounted for a substantial portion of HCV infections in the past. Approximately 20% of cases are associated with sexual exposure either to an infected partner or multiple partners and 10% with perinatal, occupational (including hemodialysis), or household transmission. The other 10% is not known.[2,6]

4. How is HCV transmitted among injection drug users?

Transmission in injection drug users occurs through the sharing of HCV-infected syringes and needles, either directly or through contamination of drug preparation equipment. Worldwide 50–90% of injection drug abusers are infected with HCV. Use of intranasal cocaine in the absence of drug injecting has rarely been implicated in the transmission of HCV.[1,3] No data indicate that tattooing or body piercing alone is a risk factor.[1,3]

5. Discuss the transmission of HCV through unprotected sexual exposure.

Unprotected sexual contacts of people who have a history of HCV infection and people who have been exposed to more than two sexual partners are at risk of acquiring HCV. There appears to be a lower prevalence of HCV with long-term spouses (1.5%) who have chronic HCV infection if no other risk factors for HCV infection are present. Some data indicate that sexual transmission of HCV is more efficient from males to females.[1,2] HCV infection is not substantially higher in men who have sex with men than in the heterosexual population.[1,3]

6. How is HCV transmitted perinatally?

The only constant associated with perinatal transmission is the presence of HCV RNA at the time of birth. Few researchers have studied the relationship between delivery mode and transmission, but at present there seems to be no difference in infection rates between infants delivered vaginally and infants delivered by cesarean section. Transmission through breast milk has not been documented.[1,3] The risk for acquiring infection through the perinatal route is lower for HCV than HIV. However, perinatal transmission of HCV is three times higher for mothers coinfected with HIV and HCV compared with mothers infected with HCV alone.[6]

7. Discuss the occupational transmission of HCV.

Unlike hepatitis B, HCV is not transmitted efficiently through occupational exposures to blood. The average incidence of hepatitis C antibody after an accidental percutaneous exposure is 1.8%. Transmission rarely occurs through mucous membranes to blood. No transmission has occurred through intact or nonintact skin exposures to mucus in health care workers.[1,3] Poor infection control techniques in hemodialysis units have been cited as causes for HCV transmission.[1,3]

8. How is HCV transmitted among household contacts?

Some studies have indicated an association between nonsexual contact and HCV infection. Transmission is thought to occur by direct or inapparent percutaneous or mucosal exposure to blood or body fluids.[1,3]

9. Describe the natural history of HCV infection.

The onset of HCV infection is often unrecognized because most patients are asymptomatic and have a mild clinical course. HCV may be transmitted during the acute stage. Jaundice occurs in 20–30% of people with HCV, and 10% may have nonspecific symptoms, including anorexia, malaise, or abdominal pain. Clinical manifestations usually occur within 6–7 weeks after exposure to HCV. The average time for seroconversion is 8–9 weeks. Acute infection can be detected by an HCV RNA serologic test in 3 weeks. Within an average of 50 days virtually all patients develop cell injury. After the acute stage, 15–25% of HCV infections seem to resolve spontaneously, with no appearance of HCV RNA in serum.[1,3,6]

Chronic hepatitis C is usually not recognized until blood donor screening or when elevated levels of alanine aminotransferase (ALT), a liver enzyme, are detected during routine physical exams. The remaining 75–85% of acutely infected patients develop chronic, persistent viremia and often have fluctuating ALT elevations, indicating active liver disease. At any one time one-half of chronically infected persons may have normal ALT levels. The course of chronic disease is insidious, progressing at a slow rate. Most chronic infections lead to hepatitis and to some degree of fibrosis. Cirrhosis develops in about 20% of infected people over a period of 20–30 years. Severe complications and death occur in some persons with cirrhosis. After cirrhosis has developed, the rate of progression to liver failure and heptocellular carcinoma is 2–4%.[1,3,8]

10. What are the current diagnostic and screening tests for hepatitis C?

An **enzyme immunoassay (EIA)** for antibodies to HCV (anti-HCV) should be the initial test for diagnosis of hepatitis C. EIAs detect anti-HCV but do not distinguish among acute, chronic, and resolved infections. There are three consecutive versions of the EIA, with each version increasing in sensitivity. The third-generation EIA should be used for screening HIV-positive people; the third-generation EIA provides the best sensitivity for antibodies. The first two versions may give false-negative results because coinfected patients may lose antibodies over time.[6] If the patient is severely immunocompromised (CD4 < 100 cells/mm[3]), the polymerase chain reaction (PCR) may be needed to confirm viremia. EIA tests usually can detect antibodies within 4–10 weeks.[7] EIAs are generally inexpensive and suitable for screening both low- and high-prevalence populations. EIA sensitivity in the high-risk population has been established. A patient who has risk factors for hepatitis C and abnormal liver functions may not need supplemental testing. If a patient has no risk factors and a negative EIA test, HCV infection may be ruled out. A positive test indicates the presence of viremia and infectivity unless proved otherwise. Because anti-HCV does not appear in the serum for an average of 4–10 weeks after exposure,[7] patients with negative serologic results who appear to have viral hepatitis should be retested in 4–6 weeks.[1,3,8]

Recombinant immunoblot assays (RIAs) are used to confirm the diagnosis for a patient with normal liver enzymes when no risk factors are present. RIAs are used when the diagnosis of hepatitis C is in question because the patient has autoimmune hepatitis or hypergammaglobulinemia.[1,3,8]

HCV RNA polymerase chain reaction (PCR) detects the presence of the virus. PCR is frequently used to determine whether the virus has cleared or infection persists. Anti-HCV does not confer immunity; therefore, when patients clear the virus, they can become reinfected. Spontaneous clearance of the virus is rare once chronic infection takes place.[1,3,8]

11. What is the role of liver biopsy?

Liver biopsy can determine the activity and extent of liver damage and is the gold standard for assessment of patients with chronic hepatitis.[9] It also confirms coexisting liver diseases. Biopsy not only determines disease activity and severity but also provides an assessment for the baseline of liver damage. Liver histology is not an indicator of the ultimate disease course. The lack of alternative therapies for patients with HIV-HCV coinfection and decompensating liver disease emphasizes the need for early diagnosis and interventions with antiviral therapy for HCV infection in patients with HIV.

12. Are screening tests reliable for disease progression?

Unfortunately, reliable markers for disease outcome are not available. Currently available laboratory tests are not exact indicators of disease progression. Neither ALT elevation nor the HCV RNA level appears to be closely associated with the outcome of disease, unlike the HIV RNA level, which is highly correlated with HIV disease.[1,3]

13. What factors enhance disease progression?

Male gender, acquisition of HCV after the age of 40 years, and alcohol consumption greater than 50 gm/day can be predictors of progressive fibrosis.[6] Alcohol intake increases the rate of fibrosis in patients with HCV infection, especially those coinfected with HIV.

14. What is the effect of HIV infection on HCV progression?

HIV coinfection is an important factor in HCV disease progression. HIV infection is associated with higher HCV RNA levels and may impair the clearance of HCV in acutely infected patients, resulting in increased risk of chronic disease. HIV accelerates the natural history of HCV, increasing the rate at which complications develop. The prevalence of extensive disease, liver fibrosis, and moderate or severe activity is significantly higher in coinfected patients.[5] Data suggest that chronic HCV infection acts as an opportunistic pathogen in HIV-infected persons, since both the incidence and severity are increased. HCV has been included in the *Guidelines for the*

Prevention of Opportunistic Infections in Persons Infected with Human Immunodeficiency since 1999. However, HCV is not considered an AIDS-defining illness.[4,5]

15. What is the treatment during the acute phase of the disease?

No studies have evaluated the treatment of acute disease. Some studies outside the United State have shown that monotherapy with interferon may be associated with a higher rate of re-solved infection. Treatment started early in the course of chronic HCV infection may be as effec-tive as treatment started during the acute phase. However, because HCV infection spontaneously resolves in 15–25% of patients, it may be unnecessary to expose them to the side effects of an-tiviral therapy. Therefore, treatment is focused at the chronic phase of the disease.[1,3,5,6]

16. Discuss the treatment for chronic HCV liver disease.

Treatment is recommended for patients with chronic HCV who are at greatest risk for pro-gression to cirrhosis, including anti-HCV–positive persons with elevated liver enzymes, detectable HCV RNA, or a liver biopsy that indicates portal or bridging fibrosis or at least moderate degrees of inflammation and necrosis. Two different drug regimens have been approved in the United States for hepatitis C: monotherapy with alpha interferon and combination therapy with alpha in-terferon and ribavirin. Among patients without HIV coinfection, both approaches may yield a vi-rologic response. Different HCV genotypes have different response rates to antiviral therapy. Rates of response in patients infected with genotype 1 (the most common genotype in the United States) is generally lower than in patients with other genotypes and may require a longer period of treatment. Therefore, recommendations should be based on the HCV genotype and viral load. Combination therapy is associated with more side effects than monotherapy, but combination ther-apy is preferable. Even if no virologic response is initiated, alpha interferon may lower the risk of progression to hepatocellular carcinoma in HCV-infected patients with cirrhosis. Monotherapy is reserved for patients with a contraindication to ribavirin. Treatment is based on the 1999 HCV consensus guidelines, suggesting that previously untreated persons without contraindications to interferon or ribavirin should receive combination therapy. Interferon with an attachment of a glycol (pegulated interferon) results in a higher rate of response than conventional monotherapy with alpha interferon.[6,7] Clinical studies are ongoing to assess the role of the combination of peg-interferon and ribavirin.[6]

For persons coinfected with HIV and HCV, monotherapy appears to be well tolerated, al-though the response rate varies. Combination therapy should increase the rates of response in coinfected persons, but the long-term effects of combination therapy in coinfected patients have not been studied thoroughly. Random trials to evaluate long-term effects of combination drugs are presently under way to clarify the role of combination therapy in coinfected patients. The in-creased side effects of combination therapy may decrease the patient's morale and compromise adherence and/or lead to negative outcomes.

17. Are patients with HCV infection candidates for liver transplantation?

Patients with HCV infection alone and decompensated cirrhosis and some patients with early hepatocellular carcinoma are candidates for liver transplantation. Because few liver transplants are done in patients with HIV-HCV coinfection, data reflecting outcome are not available.

18. Should immune globulin be given for postexposure management of hepatitis C?

The Advisory Committee on Immunization Practices concluded that immune globulin is not indicated for postexposure prophylaxis.[4] No data indicate that treatment is more effective during the acute phase of infection than during the chronic stage. Assessments have not been made of postexposure use of antiviral agents. Early initiation of interferon is associated with a higher rate of the resolved infections, but interferon has not been approved for use in the acute phase of hepatitis C. Some preliminary evidence has been associated with improved patient outcomes.[4]

19. Describe the postexposure follow-up of health care, emergency medical, and public safety workers.

Postexposure follow-up testing needs include the source (person) who may have the disease and the person exposed to that source.

- **For the source:** baseline testing for anti-HCV
- **For the person exposed to an HCV-positive source:** baseline and follow-up testing, including baseline testing for anti-HCV and ALT level and activity and follow-up testing at 4–6 months for anti-HCV and ALT liver activity.
- **Confirmation:** by supplemental anti-HCV testing of all anti-HCV results reported as positive by enzyme immunoassay.[5]

20. What are the primary prevention strategies for HCV?

Primary prevention aims to reduce the risk for contracting HCV infection. Good hand hygiene and standard precautions should be used in all health care settings for all patients. Primary prevention for injection drug use should eliminate the chief route of transmission. Injection drug abusers should be advised to stop using illicit drugs and to enter and complete substance abuse treatment, including relapse prevention programs. People who continue to use drugs should be taught never to reuse or share syringes, to use only syringes from a reliable source, to use new sterile syringes to prepare and inject drugs, to use a new or disinfected container, to clean the injection site with alcohol, and to dispose of syringes safely after one use. They should be vaccinated against hepatitis A and B.

Although intranasal cocaine use has been rarely implicated, HIV-infected people who continue to use drugs intranasally should be advised not to share equipment. No data indicate that exposure to tattooing or body piercing increases risk of HCV infection, but the potential risk for infection is high if proper techniques have not been used. Safer sexual practices include the use of condoms during sexual activity. In households that include someone diagnosed with HCV, sharing of razors or toothbrushes should be avoided.[1,3,5,8,9]

21. What are the secondary prevention strategies for HCV?

Secondary prevention reduces the risks of liver and other chronic diseases in HCV-infected persons. Populations or persons who should be tested routinely for HCV include users of illegal injection drugs, prior recipients of transfusions or organ transplants, people who had medical conditions such as long-term hemodialysis or received clotting factor concentrates produced before 1987, and people with persistently abnormal ALT levels. Others who should be routinely tested for HCV include health care, emergency, and public safety workers after needlesticks, sharps or mucosal exposures to HCV-positive blood and children born to HCV-positive mothers.[1,3,6,9]

22. What is the likely future of HCV infection worldwide?

If trends continue, HCV will continue to have a major effect globally. The high rate of progression from acute to chronic disease shows that HCV remains different from other viral hepatitis. New therapeutic approaches, new communicative models to deliver preventive messages, development of a vaccine, and new antivirals will decrease the incidence of this challenging virus.

BIBLIOGRAPHY

1. Centers for Disease Control and Prevention: Recommendations for prevention and control of hepatitis C virus (HCV) infection and HCV-related chronic disease. MMWR 47(RR-19):1–39, 1998.
2. Centers for Disease Control and Prevention: 1999 USPHS/IDSA guidelines for the prevention of opportunistic infections with human immunodeficiency virus: U. S. Public Health Service (USPHS) and Infectious Diseases Society of America (IDSA). MMWR 48(RR-10), 1999.
3. Centers for Disease Control and Prevention: Recommendations for prevention and control of hepatitis C virus (HCV) infection and HCV-related chronic disease. What clinicians and other health professionals need to know. 2001. Available at http://www.cdc.gov.

4. Centers for Disease Control and Prevention: Updated U. S. guidelines for the management of occupational exposures to HBV, HCV, and HIV and recommendations for postexposure prophylaxis. MMWR 50(RR-11):1–52, 2001.
5. Centers for Disease Control and Prevention: Most frequently asked questions and answers about coinfection with HIV and hepatitis C virus. 2001. Available at http://www.cdc.gov/hepatitis.
6. Expert Perspectives: Strategies for the management of HIV/HCVcoinfection II. 2001. Available at http://www.projectsinknowledge.com/hiv-hcv/index.html.
7. Lauer GM, Walker BD: Hepatitis C virus infection. N Engl J Med 345:41–52, 2001.
8. Proceedings of the National Institute of Health consensus Development Conference (1997). Management of hepatitis C. Hepatology 26(Suppl 1). Available at http://www.hepnet.com/nihstate.htm.
9. Sulkowski MS, Mast EE, Seeff LB, Thomas DL: Hepatitis C virus infection as an opportunistic disease in persons infected with human immunodeficiency virus. Clin Infect Dis 30 (Suppl 1):S77–S84, 2000.
10. Thomas D, et al: The natural history of hepatitis C virus infection. Host , viral, and environmental factors. JAMA 284:450–456, 2000.

12. OPPORTUNISTIC INFECTIONS

Judy K. Shaw, MS, ACRN, ANP-C

Opportunistic infections (OIs) remain a significant cause of morbidity and mortality for people with HIV/AIDS. Nurses can intervene by educating clients about medications and adherence as well as precautions to help reduce the risk of infection. In addition, a careful health history and physical examination focused on symptoms specifically related to OIs can facilitate early detection and positive outcomes.

1. What is an OI?

Think of the body as a carefully balanced system of positive and negative forces. In a healthy person the forces balance perfectly, allowing each system to work efficiently. This balanced state is called homeostasis. When one system fails for any reason, the balance shifts. This is basically what happens when a patient with HIV/AIDS develops an OI. The immune system, made up of different types of white blood cells that protect the body from infective organisms, is no longer able to maintain control, allowing fungi, protozoa, bacteria, and viruses to invade the body and cause illness. Many of the infective organisms are natural flora in the body and perform an important part in maintaining homeostasis when present in proper numbers. For example, bacteria that are present in the bowel help to break down nutrients but can cause illness (diarrhea, gas, bloating) if they are allowed to multiply out of control. In addition, some organisms that are native to a particular environment infect the majority of inhabitants. If a person with an intact immune system becomes infected with one of these organisms, he or she may experience mild-to-moderate symptoms, develop antibodies, and recover fully. If the person's immune system is not intact, he or she can become seriously ill and may even die.

2. What group of people is most likely to become infected with OIs?

For OIs to invade the body and cause illness, the immune system must not be working properly. Immunosuppression, or immune compromise as it is also called, can occur for a variety of reasons, including, but not limited to, chronic disease, advanced age, organ transplants, chemotherapy for cancer, and HIV/AIDS. Immunosuppression that is chemically induced may reverse itself once the medication is stopped.

3. Does everyone with HIV/AIDS get an OI?

Not everyone with HIV/AIDS is infected with an OI. It is important to understand that a positive HIV status refers to infection with the human immunodeficiency virus. Seropositive people are less likely than a person with AIDS to become infected with an OI because their immune system is usually more intact. Having AIDS means that the CD4 lymphocyte count is 200 mm^3 or less or that the person has (or has had) an AIDS-defining illness. The terms HIV and AIDS are a way to stage the disease and to assess its progression. Without effective treatment HIV progresses to AIDS. As the CD4 count becomes lower in the natural progression of the disease, the likelihood of developing an OI becomes greater.

Earlier in the AIDS pandemic, before effective antiretroviral therapy was available, OIs were the number-one cause of morbidity and mortality among persons with AIDS. In fact, the Centers for Disease Control and Prevention (CDC) have categorized certain OIs as AIDS-defining illnesses. With the advent of highly active antiretroviral therapy (HAART), the number of cases of OIs has decreased significantly, and use of effective therapy is now the best approach to prevention.[9] In addition, improvements in chemoprophylaxis for OIs (medications taken to prevent infection) have also reduced the incidence in people with AIDS. The most likely reasons for OIs to occur now are nonadherence to therapy (either HAART or OI prophylaxis) or failure to respond to HAART.

4. What are the most common causes of OIs?

Fungi, protozoa, bacteria, and viruses can cause OIs. OIs can infect almost every system in the body. They have many different presenting symptoms and may look quite different in their presentation from person to person. Some OIs are easier to diagnose than others, and many share the same or similar symptoms, making an accurate diagnosis difficult. Only certain OIs are spread by person-to-person contact.

5. What are some of the most common OIs caused by fungi?

Fungi, like other organisms, can cause infection and illness when the natural host defense system is unable to prevent invasion. The most common OIs caused by fungi in this setting are candidiasis, histoplasmosis, aspergillosis, and coccidioidomycosis. All of these fungi are found naturally in the environment and become a threat only when the host is immunocompromised.

6. What is candidiasis?

Thrush is the common name for oral candidiasis. The oral cavity is only one area of the body that can be infected by fungi. Candidiasis results from fungal invasion of mucosal surfaces and skin. *Candida albicans* is the candidal species most often identified as the causative agent of these infections. *C. albicans* is found abundantly in the environment and is also part of the normal body flora. It most commonly infects the oral, esophageal, or vaginal mucosa. Presenting symptoms include white patches that can cause pain and/or difficulty with swallowing in the mouth or esophagus and burning, pain, erythema, and itching of the vagina. In severe immuno-suppression, invasive systemic fungal infection can occur. The most common presenting symptom is fever. Other *Candida* species are more likely responsible when dissemination occurs.[8]

7. How is candidiasis diagnosed?

Diagnosis of oral and vaginal candidiasis is often made on clinical appearance but can be verified by microscopic examination of a scraping of the lesion using 10% potassium hydroxide (KOH). Visualization of yeast and pseudohyphae is a positive finding. Esophageal candidiasis is also usually diagnosed based on clinical findings and history. It occurs most often in the presence of oral lesions and symptoms that include dysphagia (difficulty with swallowing) and/or odynophagia (painful swallowing). If there is no improvement with treatment, more invasive testing, such as endoscopy or biopsy, is recommended to rule out other pathogens.

8. What treatment is recommended for candidiasis?

Treatment varies, depending on the location of infection. Prophylaxis is not recommended unless the patient has severe recurrent episodes because of the low mortality associated with oropharyngeal and vaginal candidiasis. In addition, treatment of only acute episodes limits the likelihood of fungal resistance development.

Oral	Clotrimazole troche, 10 mg 5 times daily *or*
	Nystatin, 100,000 u/ml oral suspension, 5 ml gargled 5 times/day
	(Either of these medications should be used until symptoms resolve)
	or
	Fluconazole, 100 mg/day × 10–14 days
Esophageal	Fluconazole, 200–400 mg/day × 7–14 days *or*
	Itraconazole, 200–400 mg/day × 7–14 days *or*
	Amphotericin B, 0.3–0.5 mg/kg IV
Vaginal	Clotrimazole, 1% cream at bedtime × 7–14 nights *or*
	Terconazole cream intravaginally, 40 mg at bedtime × 3 nights *or*
	Fluconazole, 150 mg, 1 dose

9. What causes histoplasmosis?

Histoplasmosis results from infection with *Histoplasma capsulatum*, another fungus that causes disease in people who are immunocompromised. It is found in soil contaminated by bird and bat manure. Some geographic areas are more endemic than others, including the South

Central and Midwestern United States, South America, Central America, and the Caribbean. Infection occurs when spores are inhaled. Acute presentations of histoplasmosis may be due to new infection or reactivation of latent disease when CD4 counts fall below 100 mm³.

10. What are the symptoms of histoplasmosis? How is it diagnosed?

Fever and cough are the most common presentations of histoplasmosis. With pneumonitis, chest x-rays may show diffuse bilateral interstitial infiltrates, but radiographic findings are not always reliable because of many false-negative results.[8] Disseminated disease is common; signs and symptoms include fatigue, weight loss, nausea, diarrhea, and hepatosplenomegaly. In such patients infection may result in encephalitis, focal brain lesions, or sepsis. A diagnosis can be made by cultures from blood, lesions, bone marrow, urine, or liver samples positive for *H. capsulatum*.

11. Summarize the treatment for histoplasmosis.

Treatment for acute disease differs according to the severity of the presenting symptoms.

Mild symptoms   Itraconazole, 200 mg 3 times/day for 3 days and then 2 times/day for 12 weeks

Severe symptoms   Amphotericin B, 0.7–1 mg/kg/day IV × 3–14 days *or* Lipid formulation of amphotericin B, 3 mg/kg/day IV × 3–14 days

Current recommendations are for patients to remain on suppressive therapy for life once they have had an acute episode of histoplasmosis. There is insufficient evidence to determine whether increases in CD4 cells after initiation of HAART result in a lower incidence of disease reactivation.[9]

Maintenance therapy Itraconazole, 200 mg 3 times/day for 3 days; then 2 times/day × 12 weeks; then once daily.

Prophylaxis with itraconazole, 200 mg 2 times/day, is recommended only for people with CD4 less than 100 mm³ who live in hyperendemic areas or who are at an especially high risk of infection because of occupational exposure.[9]

12. What is aspergillosis?

Aspergillus species are found in soil and on stored or decaying vegetation in all parts of the world and are usually acquired through inhalation. *A. fumigatus* and *A. flavus* are the most common species responsible for infection in humans.[5] Although the portal of entry into the body is through the lungs, infection can also occur in other parts of the body, including the external ear, paranasal sinuses, heart, and skin. The immunocompromised status of the person, rather than length or quantity of fungus involved in the exposure, is the greatest risk factor for infection.

13. How is aspergillosis diagnosed?

Positive cultures for *Aspergillus* should not always be taken at face value because the organism can grow freely in labs and is often a common contaminant. In addition, positive cultures may result from colonization rather than acute infection. Client history, immune status, and clinical findings are often relied on for a presumptive diagnosis. A definitive diagnosis depends on demonstration that the organism is invading tissue[7] or the presence of an aspergilloma (fungal ball) on radiographic imaging of the lungs or sinuses.

14. How is aspergillosis treated?

Intravenous amphotericin B remains the first-line treatment for invasive aspergillosis. Alternatively, clients who are unable to tolerate the nephrotoxic effects that may result as a side effect of amphotericin B can be treated with liposomal amphotericin B. Itraconazole, following a course of IV amphotericin B or as monotherapy, may also be prescribed for nonmeningeal infections. In severe cases, surgical removal of infected tissue, heart valve, or aspergilloma may be necessary, along with medication to increase the likelihood of a successful outcome. In cases of severe immunosuppression (in AIDS, CD4 < 50 mm³) prognosis is usually poor.[6] Providing psychosocial support and encouraging adherence to HAART therapy are key areas for nurses caring for clients with *Aspergillus* infection.

15. What is coccidioidomycosis?

Coccidioidomycosis is a fungal infection that results from infection with *Coccidioides immitis*. The organism is found in the soil, and, as with histoplasmosis, the route of infection is inhalation of spores found in dust. Infection usually occurs in people with a CD4 count less than 250 mm^3. Presenting symptoms are similar to a flu-like illness and include fever, fatigue, cough, and weight loss. Arid geographic locations, including Texas, Arizona, and California in the U.S. and Central and South America, are most often reported as having the greatest number of cases.

16. How is coccidioidomycosis diagnosed?

A thorough history and assessment of symptoms and clinical findings suggest infection with this organism. Usual symptoms of pulmonary infection are fever and productive cough, whereas with disseminated disease clients experience more systemic symptoms such as malaise and lymphadenopathy. Positive chest x-rays show diffuse interstitial and/or nodular infiltrates, hilar adenopathy, or pulmonary infiltrates. Calcifications and cavitations may also be seen.[4] Disseminated disease is diagnosed by positive cultures from blood, urine, or cerebrospinal fluid. Accurate diagnosis is often difficult because of the low index of suspicion for fungal disease. In addition, infection may be the result of reactivation of latent disease with deterioration of the immune system.

17. Summarize the treatment for coccidioidomycosis.

Acute treatment
- For severe disseminating disease: amphotericin B, 1.0 mg/kg once daily IV until the patient improves; then switch to treatment for mild-to-moderate disease, as listed below
- For mild-to-moderate disease: itraconazole, 400–800 mg/day, *or* fluconazole, 400–800 mg/day

Lifelong maintenance therapy is needed. At this time it is not recommended to stop therapy if CD4 counts rise after treatment with HAART.

Maintenance therapy
- Fluconazole, 400 mg/day, *or*
- Itraconazole, 400 mg/day

No treatment for prophylaxis is recommended, according to the U.S. Public Health Service and the Infectious Diseases Society of America.[9]

18. What is *Cryptococcus*?

Cryptococcus neoformans is an encapsulated fungus found in soil that has been contaminated with bird manure. Infection results after inhalation of the organism. Although the lungs are thought to be the initial portal of entry, infection spreads rapidly in an immunocompromised person, resulting in dissemination to other organs. The central nervous system (CNS) is often infected, and the resulting meningitis can be life-threatening. Infection may be acute or result from reactivation of a latent infection when the CD4 count is less than 100 mm^3.

19. Describe the symptoms of cryptococcal infection. How is it diagnosed?

Clients with cryptococcal meningitis present with symptoms that mimic other diseases: headache, gait disturbances, irritability, nausea, and confusion. Almost one-third of patients have papilledema, swelling, and inflammation of the optic nerve.[2] Cryptococcal meningitis is usually diagnosed by examination of the cerebrospinal fluid (CSF) obtained via lumbar puncture for cryptococci or cryptococcal antigen. To confirm cryptococci as the causative agents for pneumonia, bronchial alveolar lavage (BAL) fluid is examined for organisms. In disseminated disease a positive blood or tissue culture is confirmatory. Pulmonary infection results in a high incidence of chest pain and usually appears as dense infiltrates on chest x-ray. As for other fungal infections, amphotericin B is the first-line therapy for severe infection, followed with oral azole therapy for suppression. Flucytosine has been used as adjunctive therapy, but side effects make its effectiveness questionable.

20. What OIs do protozoa cause?

Protozoa and cytomegalovirus (CMV) are the most common causes of chronic diarrhea in persons with HIV/AIDS.[4] Protozoa are transmitted via the oral-fecal route or may be spread through ingestion of contaminated water and/or food and by person-to-person contact. Oocysts are excreted by infected people or animals that contaminate the soil and introduce the protozoa into the food cycle. Infection can also be spread among homosexual men who engage in anal intercourse. Like fungi, these protozoa are ubiquitous in the environment and, except in cases of immunosuppression, people who become infected remain asymptomatic or have only mild symptoms. The most common protozoa that cause infection in persons with HIV/AIDS are *Cryptosporidium parvum* (cryptosporidiosis), *Isospora belli* (isosporiasis), *Microsporidia* (microsporidiosis), and *Toxoplasma gondii* (toxoplasmosis).

21. What are the symptoms of diarrhea caused by protozoa? How can the causative agent be identified?

Protozoa usually infect the small bowel or portions of the colon, causing voluminous diarrhea that is watery but without blood. After a 7–10 day incubation period, symptoms may include cramping, abdominal discomfort, and anorexia. Severe chronic diarrhea leads to malabsorption, weight loss, and wasting. Diagnosis is made by identification of the organism from stool samples or tissue biopsy.

22. Discuss the treatment for diarrhea caused by protozoa.

There are no treatment recommendations for diarrhea caused by protozoa. Prevention is the best treatment. People with HIV/AIDS should be advised to avoid drinking water from dug wells, streams, or lakes. When contamination in municipal water supplies is suspected, the recommendation to boil water for one full minute should be observed.[9] Because freezing does not reduce the possibility of infection, only ice cubes made from filtered or boiled water should be considered safe. Fruit juice and dairy products that are not pasteurized should also be avoided.

People with HIV/AIDS should be cautioned not to adopt a young or stray animal as a pet. They should avoid animal yards contaminated with feces and never care for or bring home a pet that has diarrhea. Only healthy pets 1 year of age or older should be considered for adoption. If there is any reason to suspect that the pet is not healthy, stools can be examined for protozoa by a veterinarian. Hand-washing is an essential means of preventing infection.

Symptomatic treatment consists of fluid and electrolyte replacement and antimotility therapy, such as loperamide or tincture of opium. Dietary modifications include avoidance of fatty food, caffeine, and dairy products. There are anecdotal accounts of improvement with the use of paromomycin, azithromycin, metronidazole, and trimethoprim/sulfamethoxazole. Increases in CD4 count have also been associated with improvement of protozoan infection.[10]

23. Do protozoa and parasites cause only diarrhea?

Although many protozoa and parasites affect mainly the gastrointestinal system, some organisms infect other parts of the body. For example, toxoplasmosis infects the central nervous system.

24. What is toxoplasmosis?

Toxoplasma gondii, the organism responsible for toxoplasmosis, is the primary cause of CNS lesions in advanced AIDS. Cats are the definitive hosts for *T. gondii*, which is spread to humans by the oral-fecal route either by direct handling of cat feces or ingestion of cysts in undercooked meat from infected animals. After acute infection organisms encyst and become latent. Toxoplasmosis in persons with AIDS can result from acute infection or reactivation of latent infection as the immune system deteriorates. Symptoms include headache, gait disturbances, confusion, low-grade fever, seizure activity, focal neurologic deficits, hemiparesis, and personality changes.

25. How is toxoplasmosis diagnosed?

Diagnosis may be presumptive based on the history and clinical findings, especially results of neurologic testing and assessment of CD4 count (< 100 mm^3). Improvement of symptoms after treatment is often considered to be confirmatory. A positive CT scan of the head shows hypodense lesions that enhance in a ring pattern with the use of contrast. Lesions are commonly found in the basal ganglia but also can be found in other locations of the brain. Edema may be present as well. Magnetic resonance imaging (MRI) shows localized, high-signal abnormalities.

26. Summarize the recommended treatments for toxoplasmosis.

First-line treatment Pyrimethamine, loading dose of 100–200 mg, followed by 50–100 mg/day *plus*
Folinic acid, 10 mg/day *plus*
Sulfadiazine *or* trisulfapyrimidine, 4–8 gm/day × 6 weeks
Alternative treatment Pyrimethamine, loading dose of 100–200 mg, followed by 50–70 mg/day *plus*
Folinic acid, 10 mg/day *plus* one of the following:
Clarithromycin, 1000 mg every 12 hours *or*
Azithromycin, 1200–1500 mg once daily
Lifelong maintenance therapy is recommended at this time.
Maintenance therapy Pyrimethamine, 25–75 mg/day, *plus*
Sulfadiazine, 500–1000 mg 4 times/day *plus*
Folinic acid, 10 mg/day
This is the first-line therapy for maintenance. Other options are available.
Prophylaxis Trimethoprim/sulfamethoxazole DS or SS, 1 tablet/day orally *or*
Trimethoprim/sulfamethoxazole DS, 1 tablet orally 3 times/week

27. What is PCP?

PCP was one of the first OIs associated with AIDS. Estimates of incidence rates reported before the advent of antiretroviral therapy range from 50% to 90% of the AIDS population. HIV testing after a diagnosis of PCP is standard community practice. *P. carinii* is recognized as a fungus but until recently was also considered to have characteristics of the protozoa famly.[1] *P. carinii* is found abundantly in the environment. The route of infection is thought to be airborne because the organism primarily infects the lungs. A high prevalence rate of antibodies has been identified in the general population as early as childhood, leading to the theory that the majority of cases are due to reactivation of a latent infection. People with a CD4 count less than 200 mm^3 are considered to be at risk and should receive prophylaxis.

28. How is PCP diagnosed and treated?

Symptoms of PCP can be hard to identify, especially in patients not known to be infected with HIV. The most common presenting symptoms are dyspnea, fever, and nonproductive cough. Initial symptoms may be nonspecific (e.g., intermittent fever, fatigue, malaise) but usually worsen over a period of several weeks. A positive chest x-ray shows bilateral interstitial infiltrates, but x-rays may be normal early in the disease process. Results of arterial blood gases usually indicate hypoxia, and the serum level of lactate dehydrogenase (LDH) may be elevated. Sputum cultures or specimens obtained from bronchoscopy with bronchial alveolar lavage may be needed for a definitive diagnosis.

Mild-to-moderate cases can be treated with careful monitoring in an outpatient setting, if the client adheres to the following regimen:
Outpatient treatment
Trimethoprim/sulfamethoxazole DS, 2 tablets 4 times/day
Clients who have more severe disease, who are nonadherent with medications, or who need psychosocial support can be treated on an inpatient basis with any of the following.
Inpatient treatment
Trimethoprim, 15 mg/kg/day, *plus* sulfamethoxazole, 75 mg/kg/day IV in 3–4 divided doses, *or*
Dapsone, 100 mg/day, + trimethoprim, 15 mg/kg/day × 21 days, *or*
Pentamidine, 4 mg/kg/day IV × 21 days, *or*

Clindamycin, 600 mg IV every 8 hours *plus* oral primaquine, 30 mg/day × 21 days, *or*

Atovaquone, 750 mg 2 times/day with food × 21 days

Additional alternative treatments are also available.

Lifelong maintenance therapy is recommended at this tme.

Corticosteroids should be considered in addition to the previous therapies in clients with moderate-to-severe hypoxia.

Prophylaxis is strongly recommended for people with CD4 counts less than 200 mm³. In addition, people with a CD4 T-lymphocyte percentage less than 14% or who have had an AIDS-defining illness also may be considered for prophylsxis. Prophylaxis can be discontinued in persons who are receiving effective HAART therapy after 3 months with a rise in CD4 count > 200 mm³ but should be restarted if the CD4 count falls below that value.

Prophylaxis

Trimethoprim/sulfamethoxazole DS or SS, 1 tablet daily *or*

Dapsone, 100 mg/day *or*

Aerosolized pentamidine, 300 mg monthly via nebulizer

29. What bacterial infections are common in people infected with HIV/AIDS?

People infected with HIV, especially those with AIDS, are more likely to become sick from common bacterial organisms because they do not have the natural mechanism to fight off invasion. It is important to remember that people with HIV/AIDS do not always have an exotic etiology for their disease. In fact, they are likely to be infected with the same organisms that cause illness in other members of their community.

• The most common cause of bacterial pneumonia among people with HIV/AIDS is *Streptococcus pneumoniae*. Common symptoms include fever, chills, productive cough, and shortness of breath. Diagnosis can be made by radiologic imaging, which usually shows consolidation or bilateral interstitial infiltrates, or positive blood or sputum cultures. Penicillin is often used as first-line therapy; susceptibility and resistance testing yields confirmation of the choice of medication.

• A second organism, *Haemophilus influenzae*, is often responsible for recurrent respiratory illnesses. The daily use of trimethoprim-sulfamethoxazole for PCP prophylaxis is thought to reduce the risk of developing bacterial infections as well but is not currently recommended for that purpose alone.[9]

• *Salmonella* infection usually results from ingestion of contaminated food (i.e., eggs or poultry) and/or water or from contamination due to marijuana or animals (especially chicks, ducks, turtles). Symptoms appear 6–48 hours later. Diarrhea, fever, chills, and other gastrointestinal symptoms are usually present. Diagnosis is made by culturing stools for enteric pathogens. Ciprofloxacin, 500 mg 2 times/day for 2 weeks, may be used to treat clients with HIV/AIDS. The nurse should stress the need for good handwashing techniques and the need for adequate fluid and electrolyte replacement.

• *Shigella* infection, also known as bacillary dysentery, most often results from person-to-person contact with someone who has the illness; cases associated with contaminated food and water have been reported.[5] The organism is highly virulent, and only a small number of organisms are necessary to cause illness in a host. Thus, outbreaks are common among institutionalized populations. Symptoms usually manifest 1–7 days after introduction of the organism, and clients present with mild-to-severe watery diarrhea with or without fever. Diagnosis is made by identification of enteric pathogens in stool samples. Fecal leukocytes are also a common finding. Treatment includes trimethoprim/sulfamethoxazole DS, 1 tablet 2 times/day for 3 days, or ciprofloxacin, 500 mg twice daily for 3 days.

• *Campylobacter* from undercooked poultry accounts for 50–70% of reported cases of infection,[2] but the organism may be found in other animals as well. Symptoms, which usually present 2–4 days after ingestion of contaminated food, include diarrhea, fever, and abdominal pain and cramps. Initial treatment may be supportive, including replacement of fluids and electrolytes. Erythromycin, 250 mg 4 times/day for 5–7 days, may be used if symptoms worsen. Ciprofloxacin, 500 mg twice daily for 3–5 days, is usually the alternative treatment.

30. Is tuberculosis (TB) still a problem in the U.S.?

Mycobacterium tuberculosis is the organism that causes most cases of TB. There has been an overall increase in incidence of TB in the U.S. over the past 10 years, and TB continues to be a serious problem among elderly people, poor people, immigrants, inmates, and people with HIV. In fact, by some estimates as many of 50% of patients infected with TB also have HIV/AIDS.[8] This association may be due to a number of factors, including socioeconomic factors as well as immunosuppression. People with HIV/AIDS are estimated to have a 30–40% greater chance of infection after close contact with someone who is infected than people who are not immunosuppressed.[8] In addition, an increasing number of cases of multidrug-resistant TB (MDR TB) are reported annually, leading to suspicions that the incidence rates will continue to rise.

31. How does TB infection spread? What tests are used to make a diagnosis?

TB is spread by the inhalation of aerosolized droplets expelled by an infected person during coughing, sneezing, or talking. Organisms are transported from the portal of entry in the lungs to lymph nodes and other parts of the body. Infection is classified as pulmonary (lungs only) or extrapulmonary (lungs and/or other organs). If the person's immune system is able to develop host immunity, organisms are entrapped in granulomatous lesions made up of large numbers of macrophages that migrate to the site of the infection. Once contained, organisms survive but do not spread. In such cases, disease may be reactivated by severe immunosuppression. If the system is not able to provide immunity, primary infection occurs. General symptoms include fever, weight loss, night sweats, and fatigue.

The purified protein derivative (PPD) skin test can identify active infection, even in clients who are asymptomatic. These finding are less reliable in people with HIV/AIDS, who may not be able to mount a host response. Anergy, or the inability to react to specific antigens, can lead to false-negative results. In people with HIV/AIDS, an induration > 5mm after 48–72 hours is considered a positive finding. Upper lobe infiltrates and cavitary lesions are indicative of positive results on chest x-ray. Stains for acid-fast bacillus and cultures from sputum, blood, or tissues are also diagnostic.

32. What are the current treatment recommendations for TB in people with HIV/AIDS?

Because of the increasing incidence of MDR TB, susceptibility results should be considered before any medication regimen is initiated. Four drugs are used for induction of treatment for acute TB disease; after several weeks or months, depending on the regimen chosen, treatment continues with 2 or 3 drugs. Drug–drug interactions between rifampin and protease inhibitors are common and should be avoided by the use of alternate medication. Treatment with isoniazid and pyrimethamine is recommended for clients who have a positive skin test but no additional indications of acute disease. Drug-prescribing recommendations are extensive. The most current treatment recommendations can be found in the *Morbidity and Mortality Weekly Report* (MMWR) published by the CDC.

33. Do TB and *Microbacterium avium* complex (MAC) cause the same disease?

MAC, which consists of two similar organisms (*M. avium* and *M intracellulare*), is termed nontuberculous mycobacteria. Both organisms are found abundantly in the environment and infect people with severe immune suppression (CD4 < 50 mm³). In fact, more than 40% of people with AIDS are thought to become infected at some time during their illness.[1]

Symptoms of disseminated disease include night sweats, fever, diarrhea, abdominal pain, and weight loss. Diagnosis of active disease can be made from sterile cultures identifying the organisms.

34. Summarize the treatment options for MAC.

Active disease   Clarithromycin, 500 mg twice daily, *plus* ethambutol, 15/mg/kg/day, *or* Azithromycin, 600 mg/day, *plus* ethambutol, 15 mg/kg/day *with or without* rifabutin, 300 mg/day

Treatment should continue for at least 1 year and should not be discontinued until the CD4 count is $> 100^3$ for 3–6 months and the client is asymptomatic.[1]

Prophylaxis   Azithromycin, 1200 mg once weekly, *or*
Clarithromycin, 500 mg twice daily

35. Do viruses cause the greatest number of infections in people with HIV/AIDS?

Viruses play a significant role in the morbidity of people with HIV/AIDS. Recently hepatitis C (see Chapter 11) has been identified as a cause of increased mortality in persons with HIV/AIDS. Reports of coinfection are estimated to range between 30% and 60% of the HIV/AIDS population.

36. How does cytomegalovirus (CMV) affect people with HIV/AIDS?

CMV is a serious threat to people with AIDS whose CD4 counts have fallen below 50 mm^3. About one-half of the U.S. population has antibodies for CMV. Most primary infections probably occur during childhood, and the remainder are due to sexual transmission or prolonged person-to-person contact later in life.[8] Based on such data, it appears that reactivation of latent infection during advanced deterioration of the immune system may be the primary cause of CMV disease in AIDS.

CMV retinitis is the best-known infection in people with HIV/AIDS. Clients complain of altered vision, "cotton spots," floaters, or flashing lights. Without prompt diagnosis and treatment CMV lesions enlarge and progress to widespread ocular necrosis and edema, resulting in irreversible loss of sight. Annual ophthamologic examinations that include dilatation of the eye are recommended for people with HIV; more frequent exams (every 3–6 months) are recommended for people with AIDS.

CMV can infect other organs as well and should be suspected as a possible diagnosis for pneumonitis, esophagitis, colitis, cerebral lesions, polyradiculomyelitis, and transverse myelitis. Although the incidences of these diseases are less frequent than retinitis, they pose a serious threat.

37. Summarize the treatment for CMV retinitis.

Several treatment options are recommended for CMV retinitis.

Recommended initial therapy
Intraocular ganciclovir release device every 6 months *plus* oral ganciclovir, 1.0–1.5 gm
    3 times/day with meals, *or*
Foscarnet, 60 mg/kg IV every 8 hours for 14–21 days, *or*
Foscarnet, 90 mg/kg IV every 12 hours for 14–21 days, *or*
Ganciclovir, 5 mg/kg IV twice daily for 14–21 days, *or*
Cidofovir, 5 mg/kg IV every week for 2 doses, then every 2 weeks, *plus* probenecid, 2 gm
    orally 3 hours before and 2 and 8 hours after each dose

Alternative therapy
Alternating doses or a combination of foscarnet and ganciclovir *or*
Intraocular injections of foscarnet or ganciclovir *or*
Fomiversin by intravitreal injection

Maintenance therapy
Foscarnet, 90–120 mg/kg/day IV, *or*
Ganciclovir, 5–6 mg/kg IV 5–7 days/week, *or*
Ganciclovir, 1000 mg orally 3 times/day, *or*
Cidofovir, 5 mg/kg IV every other week, *or*
Intraocular gancyclovir-release device every 6 months *plus* gancyclovir, 1 gm orally
    3 times/day

The current recommended treatments for gastrointestinal, pulmonary, or central nervous system infection are IV ganciclovir and/or foscarnet. Valganciclovir, an oral agent still considered to be an experimental treatment for CMV retinitis, has had promising results in clinical trials.[3] Early diagnosis of CMV retinitis, effective HAART, and regular screening are the best ways to prevent progression of CMV disease.

38. What other viruses are considered OIs?

Viruses Considered Opportunistic Infections by the U.S. Public Health Service and Infectious Diseases Society of America

VIRAL TYPE	ROUTE OF TRANSMISSION	SYMPTOMS	DIAGNOSIS	TREATMENT	COMMENT
Herpes simplex virus	Sexual contact	Ulcerous lesions usually found on genital, anal, or oral mucosa	Tzanck smear DFA stain Biopsy	*Acute:* Acyclovir, 400 mg 3 times/day *Suppressive:* Acyclovir, 200 mg 2 times/day	Infection can occur when no lesions are present
Varicella zoster virus (VZV)	Reactivation of latent infection Primary infection as chicken pox remains dormant in dorsal root ganglia	Superficial cutaneous pain followed by rash and vesicular lesions following dermatomes	Scrapings for VZV	Famciclovir, 500 mg every 8 hr × 7 days *or* Acyclovir, 800 mg/day × 7 days	Monitor for secondary infection Postherpetic pain may last several weeks to months
Human papilloma virus	Sexual contact	Genital warts	Biopsy of condyloma	Podophyllin 25%, applied once weekly, *or* Trichloroacetic acid 50%, every week *or* Imiquimod, 5% cream, applied topically 3 tmes/week for up to 16 weeks	Excessive disease may require surgical intervention
Kaposi's sarcoma (human herpes virus-8)	Oral, needle-sharing, semen	Lesions of differing colors, size, and shape on skin or other tissues	Biopsy of lesion	Radiation therapy, cryotherapy, or injection of lesions with chemotherapy	

DFA = direct fluorescent antibody.

BIBLIOGRAPHY

1. Bartlett J, Gallant J: 2001–2002 Medical Management of HIV Infection. Baltimore, Johns Hopkins University, Division of Infectious Diseases, 2001.
2. Braunwald E, Fauci A, Kasper D, et al (eds): Harrison's Manual of Medicine, 15th ed. New York, McGraw-Hill, 2002.

3. Curran M, Noble S: Valganciclovir. Drugs 61:1145–1150, 2001.
4. Libman H, Witzburg R: A Primary Care Manual. HIV Infection. Boston, Little, Brown, 1995.
5. Mandell G, Bennett JE, Dolin R: Mandell, Douglas and Bennett's Principles and Practice of Infectious Disease, 4th ed. New York, Churchill Livingstone, 1995.
6. Patterson TF, Kirkpatrick WR, White M, et al: Invasive aspergillosis. Disease spectrum, treatment practices, and outcomes. I3 Aspergillosis Study Group. Medicine 79:250–260, 2000.
7. Reese R, Betts R: A Practical Approach to Infectious Disease, 4th ed. Boston, Little, Brown, 1996.
8. Ropka M, Williams A: HIV Nursing and Symptom Management. Boston, Jones & Bartlett, 1998.
9. U.S. Publich Health Service, Infectious Diseases Society of America: 2001 USPHS/IDSA Guidelines for the Prevention of Opportunistic Infections in Persons Infected with Human Immunodeficiency Virus. Washington, DC, U.S. Government Printing Office, 2001.
10. Vasquez E:. Opportunistic Infections. 2001. Available at http://www.thebody.com.

13. NEUROLOGIC PROBLEMS

Minda J. Hubbard, MSN, RNC, ANP

Neurologic problems are the initial manifestation of AIDS in 7–20% of cases. More than one-half of patients living with HIV experience some neurologic problem over the course of the disease. The initial presentation of the HIV-positive patient with central nervous system problems is often complex and challenging for the health care professional. This chapter provides an overview of the most common neurologic problems in caring for people with HIV/AIDS.

1. What are the most common neurologic manifestations in HIV-positive patients?

HIV-positive patients often experience illness-related problems of the central and/or peripheral nervous systems. In the central nervous system (CNS), headache and change in mental status present with the greatest frequency. In the peripheral nervous system, distal peripheral neuropathy is often encountered.

2. Describe the assessment of the HIV-positive patient complaining of headache.

The major factor to consider in the presence of headache is whether the patient has fever. If fever is present, work-up for an underlying infectious cause is needed. Depending on the level of immunosuppression (indicated by the CD4 cell count), the patient may need a full work-up for cryptococcal meningitis or toxoplasmosis, both of which require prompt medical intervention. Sinusitis is another common cause of headache and can occur at any CD4 count. Less common infectious causes of headache are syphilis, viral meningitis (including herpes and cytomegalovirus), and bacterial meningitis (including tuberculosis).[1]

If no fever is present, other causes for the headache should be considered, including tension, dental problems, allergy symptoms, migraines, and malignancy. A thorough history can often help narrow the differential diagnosis. A medication history should be included, because some medications can cause headache.

3. What factors should be considered in HIV-positive patients with mental status changes?

One of the most critical factors in assessing mental status changes is the type of onset of symptoms. In abrupt-onset mental status change, opportunistic infection must be considered, especially when the patient has fever. The most common infections of the CNS are outlined below.

Opportunistic Infections and Neoplasms of the Central Nervous System

DIAGNOSIS	CAUSE	CD4 COUNT	TREATMENT	NURSING IMPLICATIONS
Toxoplasmosis	Parasite	< 100	Pyrimethamine + folinic acid + sulfadiazine	Treatment is lifelong Monitor CBC, RFTs Encourage hydration
Cryptococcal meningitis	Fungus	< 200	Initial: amphotericin Maintenance: fluconazole (Diflucan)	Monitor BP during infusion; watch RFTs, CBC, and LFTs
PML	Virus	< 50	HAART	High mortality rate
CMV encephalitis	Virus	<50	Ganciclovir/foscarnet	High mortality rate
CNS lymphoma	Malignancy	< 100	Radiation	Treatment is palliative High mortality rate

Table continued on following page

Opportunistic Infections and Neoplasms of the Central Nervous System (Continued)

DIAGNOSIS	CAUSE	CD4 COUNT	TREATMENT	NURSING IMPLICATIONS
Neurosyphilis	Bacteria	Any	Penicillin G	Monitor RPR annually for all HIV patients
Tuberculous meningitis	Bacteria	Any	Anti-TB drugs for 12–18 mo	Monitor PPD annually for all HIV patients

CBC = complete blood count, RFTs = renal function tests, BP = blood pressure, LFTs = liver function tests, PML = progressive multifocal leukoencephalopathy, HAART = highly active antiretroviral therapy, CMV = cytomegalovirus, CNS = central nervous system, RPR = rapid plasmin reagin test, PPD = purified protein derivative test.

Bear in mind that in patients with advanced immunosuppression, fever may not always accompany infection because the patient may no longer be able to mount an immune response.

Another cause of abrupt change in mental status is metabolic abnormalities. Alterations in electrolytes and hormonal imbalance should be considered. In patients with concomitant liver disease, encephalopathy is an alteration in mental status due to elevated toxins such as ammonia. This condition can cause bouts of lethargy, confusion, and disorientation.

Medications can cause mental status changes, either by direct effect (e.g., steroid psychosis) or by drug interactions. Patients who are on highly active antiretroviral therapy (HAART) take multiple drugs metabolized in the liver. Many of these drugs alter the metabolism of other compounds in the body. Pain relievers, sedatives, and antidepressants can reach toxic levels, leading to altered mental status. Patients should be educated to inform all providers of all prescription and over-the-counter drugs that they take to facilitate close monitoring for side effects and drug interactions. Illicit drugs may also be the cause of abrupt mental status changes. Urine and serum drug toxicology screens identify this problem and help determine the appropriate treatment.

If the onset of symptoms is more gradual, the most likely cause is HIV dementia (see questions 11–13).

4. How can the CD4 count be used in determining conditions for which the patient is at risk?

The status of the immune system is a key factor in all aspects of assessing and caring for HIV-positive patients. Although some problems can manifest at any CD4 count, many are seen almost exclusively in the advanced stages of the disease. The immunocompromised patient is at risk for opportunistic infections of all kinds. When the CD4 count is below 200, risk increases for toxoplasmosis, cryptococcal meningitis, cytomegalovirus (CMV) meningitis, herpes meningitis, progressive multifocal leukoencephalopathy (PML), and CNS lymphoma. HIV-associated dementia can be encountered at higher CD4 counts, but this is quite rare. Neurologic problems that can be encountered at any CD4 count include the following:

• Neurosyphilis is a manifestation of late-stage syphilis seen in 0.5% of HIV-infected patients.
• Myopathy is disease characterized by muscle pain and weakness that usually affect the muscles of the lower extremities.
• Neuropathy is a painful and debilitating condition affecting the nerves of the feet and hands, with a variety of causes.[6]

5. How does the risk for neurologic complications change once the patient begins HAART for HIV?

The goal of HAART is to suppress HIV replication and preserve immune function. Once the immune system begins to respond favorably to a successful medication regimen, risk for opportunistic infections of all kinds is greatly reduced (particularly once the CD4 count rises over 200). A phenomenon of immune reconstitution syndrome can be encountered after successful antiretroviral treatment. As the immune system recovers function, the patient may experience reactivation of subclinical diseases previously lying dormant in the body.[5] Tuberculosis and syphilis, both potentially seen in the nervous system, have been known to flare once a patient with a previously low CD4 count begins a successful medication regimen.

6. Do antiretroviral medications have any nervous system side effects?

Several of the antivirals can cause side effects in the nervous system. Azidothymidine (AZT; Retrovir) can cause headaches, and efavirenz (Sustiva) is associated with a high incidence of dizziness, insomnia, drowsiness, vivid dreams, or difficulty with concentrating. Usually such side effects subside after the first 2–4 weeks of therapy—an important point to include in patient education.

Distal peripheral neuropathy (DPN) may be caused by d4T (Zerit), ddC (Hivid), and ddI (Videx). Patients complain of burning, tingling, shooting pains, and/or hyperesthesia or paresthesia. Symptoms usually affect the feet but can progress to the hands as well. Such symptoms can be debilitating and lead to disruption of sleep and activities of daily living, with a strong negative effect on quality of life. Patients need to be questioned about symptoms of peripheral neuropathy at every encounter.[9] Both d4T and ddI are dosed according to body weight. Always check to be sure that the patient is receiving the proper dose for her or his weight to avoid preventable drug toxicity.

7. Is it necessary to stop antiretroviral drugs when they result in DPN?

Reduced doses of d4T and ddI are sometimes sufficient to reverse DPN symptoms; if not, the drugs should be stopped before permanent damage occurs. Early intervention is the key to successful management and often leads to resolution in 4–8 weeks. However, patients should be warned that there is often a temporary increase in symptoms ("coasting period") after DPN has been identified and offending drugs have been stopped. Reassure patients that, with early intervention, symptoms usually resolve fully. If the patient has more than one risk factor for DPN, full resolution of symptoms may not be possible.[7]

8. What risk factors other than HIV can contribute to the development of DPN?

Multiple risk factors that can contribute to DPN must be considered in the assessment of the HIV-infected patient (see table below). Comorbid diabetes, vitamin B_{12} deficiency, nutritional problems, and alcoholism increase the risk for developing DPN. Advanced stage of HIV and older age are also risk factors. The patient's history should be reviewed; identification of risk factors for DPN should alert the health care provider to monitor vigilantly for onset of symptoms.

Risk Factors for Drug-related Distal Peripheral Neuropathy

Low CD4 count
Older age
Poor nutritional status
Prior nutritional status
Other medical conditions associated with DPN: diabetes, alcoholism, vitamin B_{12} deficiency
Concomitant neurotoxic agents

9. Which medications can lead to DPN?

In addition to the antiretrovirals previously mentioned, several antibacterials, drugs used in cancer treatment, and others have the potential to cause and/or exacerbate DPN symptoms.

Drugs That Can Cause or Exacerbate Peripheral Neuropathy

ANTIBACTERIALS	ANTINEOPLASTICS	ANTIRETROVIRALS	OTHER AGENTS
Dapsone	Vinblastine sulfate	d4T (Zerit)	Phenytoin
Ethionamide	Vincristine sulfate	ddC (Hivid)	Thalidomide
Isoniazid (especially if given without pyridoxine)	Cisplatin	ddI (Videx)	
Metronidazole			
Streptomycin			

10. What strategies other than eliminating offending medications can be used to manage DPN?

Adjunctive treatments can help with DPN symptom management and should always be included in the treatment plan. Neuroleptics such as gabapentin (Neurontin) and amotrigine (Lamictal), antidepressants such as amitriptyline (Elavil), and beta carotene (L-carnitor) are often effective treatment options.[7] Sometimes narcotic analgesics also are required to manage pain symptoms but should be used for short-term management only. Caution should be used with patients who have a history of substance abuse, because use of prescribed narcotics can trigger relapse.

11. Is dementia common among patients with end-stage AIDS?

The advent of successful therapies for HIV disease has resulted in a dramatic decrease in morbidity of all types. However, 15–20% of patients with advanced immunosuppression exhibit HIV-associated dementia (HAD).[9] Symptoms have an insidious onset and are exhibited as cognitive, motor, and/or behavioral changes (see table below). In addition to having a tremendous negative impact on quality of life, HAD is an independent predictor of mortality.[8]

Presenting symptoms of HIV-associated Dementia

DOMAIN	SYMPTOMS	SIGNS
Cognitive	Poor concentration Forgetfulness	Slowed mentation Poor memory, calculations
Motor	Clumsiness Unsteady gait	Slowed fine finger movements Ataxic gait
Behavioral	Lack of interest in friends and hobbies	Apathy and pseudodepression

12. What causes HAD?

HAD is an indirect result of HIV infection. The HIV virus enters the brain early in the course of disease but does not directly affect the neurons. Rather, the target cells are brain phagocytes that, when infected, produce neurotoxic secretory products. The result is inflammation and damage to the blood-brain barrier, which lead to metabolic encephalopathy and destruction of neurons.[9]

13. How is HAD treated?

Although no definitive recommendation has been made, it is generally believed that a successful HAART regimen offers protection against—and sometimes yields improvement in—HAD. Not all antiretroviral medications penetrate well into the central nervous system.

There are three classes of antiretroviral medications. Protease inhibitors are highly protein-bound and, as a result, do not cross the blood-brain barrier significantly. Among the nucleoside reverse transcriptase inhibitors (NRTIs), the only drug with demonstrated clinical evidence of reaching the nervous system is AZT (Retrovir). Other NRTIs have variable rates of penetration. In the nonnucleoside reverse transcriptase class of drugs, nevirapine (Viramune) also penetrates into the CNS fairly well. It is believed that as long as the treatment regimen includes at least one of these drugs, there will be sufficient penetration to the viral sanctuary in the brain.[2]

BIBLIOGRAPHY

1. Bartlett JG, Gallant JE: Medical Management of HIV Infection. Baltimore, Port City Press, 2000.
2. Kolson D, et al: The effects of human immunodeficiency virus in the central nervous system. Adv Virus Res 50: 2–19,1998.
3. McArthur JC: Neurology update. Hopkins HIV Rep 3:2, 1999.
4. Price RW: Neurologic disease. In Dolan R, et al (eds): AIDS Therapy. Philadelphia, Churchill Livingstone, 1999, pp. 620–638.
5. Price RW, et al: Neurological outcomes in late HIV infection: Adverse impact of neurological impairment on survival and protective effect of antiviral therapy. AIDS 13:1677–1684, 1999.

6. Roullet E: Opportunistic infections of the central nervous system during HIV-1 infection. J Neurol 246:237–243, 1999.
7. Simpson D: Update on Neurologic Complications of HIV. Volume 1: Diagnosing and Managing Peripheral Neuropathies. New York, Bristol Myers Squibb, 2000.
8. Simpson D: Update on Neurologic Complications of HIV. Volume 2: Selected Central Nervous System Disorders—Dementia, PML and Myelopathy. New York, Bristol Myers Squibb, 2000.
9. Swindells S, et al: HIV-associated dementia: New insights into disease pathogenesis and therapeutic interventions. AIDS Patient Care STDs 13(3):153–163, 1999.
10. Wright D, et al: Central nervous system opportunistic infections. Neuroimag Clin North Am 7:513–525, 1997.

14. WASTING SYNDROME AND METABOLIC AND MORPHOLOGIC COMPLICATIONS

Brian D. Arey, MSN, ANP-BC

1. What is the difference between wasting and metabolic-morphologic complications?
Wasting involves lean tissue, whereas morphologic complications involve adipose tissues. **Wasting** is involuntary weight loss with lean tissue depletion and is frequently associated with fever and chronic diarrhea. It was one of the first AIDS-defining complications and is frequently responsible for AIDS-related stigma and mortality. Wasting gave AIDS its early name in Africa: "slim disease."[21] It is more prevalent in people with untreated or advanced AIDS and may be the first AIDS-defining condition in some patients. Wasting may or may not be outwardly apparent. It can be episodic. Muscle wasting tends to occur during acute opportunistic infections and then to be replaced with fat mass once the infection has resolved. The fat may disguise the obvious signs of wasting without providing a health advantage to the patient. Loss of body cell mass equal to or greater than 45% is a stronger predictor of AIDS-related death than the CD4+ T cell count.[8,9,23]

Metabolic and morphologic complications began to be noticed around 1997, after the introduction of protease inhibitors (PIs) and the widespread use of highly active antiretroviral therapy (HAART), triple-combination antiretroviral therapy.[2] Because of this temporal correlation, HAART was the immediate suspect.[6] However, further investigation has indicated a more complicated etiology, including factors related to HIV infection itself and host genetic factors. Despite the term *lipodystrophy syndrome*, metabolic and morphologic complications are a group of symptoms with varying degrees of association that may or may not be part of a single clinical syndrome. Examples include body habitus changes (peripheral fat wasting and fat redistribution), dyslipidemia, disorders of glucose metabolism, and possibly lactic acidosis/acidemia and osteoporosis/osteopenia. Defining and determining causes of metabolic and morphologic abnormalities are difficult because any given patient may have a combination of symptoms and is unlikely to have all of them. Some patients have none of the symptoms.

2. What is lipodystrophy?
Lipodystrophy is the subcategory of morphologic complications that includes fat wasting (lipoatrophy) and fat accumulation or redistribution (lipohypertrophy). A comparison of wasting and morphologic complications is presented below

Comparison of Wasting and Morphologic Complications

PARAMETER	WASTING	LIPOATROPHY	LIPOHYPERTROPHY	FAT MALDISTRIBUTION
Body component affectged	Lean (muscle) tissue	Fat (adipose) tissue	Fat (adipose) tissue	Fat (adipose) tissue
Weight change (loss)	±	±	±	±
Generally early vs. late in disease course	Late	Early/late	Early/late	Early/late
Associated with OIs	+	±	±	±
Associated with high HIV RNA	+	±	±	±
Associated with low CD4+ T cells	+	±	±	±
Associated with HAART	—	+	+	+

OIs = opportunistic infections, HAART = highly active antiretroviral therapy.

3. What causes HIV-related wasting?

Wasting has two broad components: starvation and cachexia. **Starvation** is caused by decreased nutritional intake or malabsorption. Decreased intake may result from the decreased availability of food due to economic factors, the inability to prepare food and feed oneself, or the inability to swallow because of conditions such as esophageal candidiasis. Malabsorption may be caused by HIV, an opportunistic gastrointestinal disorder, or any diarrheal condition that speeds the passage of nutrients through the alimentary canal and reduces the ability of the body to absorb the nutrients. In starvation states, the body adapts to decreased energy intake by reducing the metabolic rate. The body catabolizes fat stores first in an attempt to preserve protein stores. Starvation may be reversed with adequate nutrition or the correction of the underlying condition causing malabsorption.

Cachexia is an acute-phase immune response to infectious or neoplastic conditions, mediated by inflammatory immune system chemical messengers known as cytokines. In cachexia, catabolic reactions exceed anabolic processes, proteolysis (the breakdown of body proteins for energy) occurs, and a net protein deficit results in the loss of lean body mass. This type of wasting is responsible for acute episodes of rapid weight loss associated with the presence of opportunistic infections.[11,12] In Africa, disseminated tuberculosis is one of the most common infections associated with wasting. Therefore, in cachexia the underlying condition must be treated; otherwise, the addition of nutrition will result in fat repletion without lean tissue repletion.

Which of these two components is responsible for weight loss in AIDS wasting syndrome remains controversial, and this controversy is reflected in the multiple factors and complex interrelationship between the two that characterize AIDS wasting.[1] For instance, reduced nutrient intake may result from factors such as lack of available food (starvation state) or anorexia caused by an illness (cachexia). The table below summarizes factors related to wasting in persons with HIV infection.

Factors Related to Wasting in HIV-Infection

Reduced nutrient intake
   Anorexia
      • Cytokine-mediated appetite suppression
      • Adverse effects of medications: nausea, vomiting, diarrhea
      • Depression
      • Social isolation
   Opportunistic infections: dysphagia, odynophagia
   Dementia
   Fatigue
   Financial hardship

Malabsorption
   HIV enteropathy
   Immunosuppression
   Opportunistic gastrointestinal infections
   Diarrhea
   Decreased intestinal transit time

Altered metabolism
   Futile cycling of energy substrates
   Increased metabolic demands
   Muscle catabolism
   Increased energy expenditure
   Decreased testosterone levels

Decreased physical activity
   Deconditioning   Anorexia
   Muscle atrophy   Diarrhea
   Fatigue   Adverse effects of medication
   Fever

4. How can nurses help patients conserve energy?

Opportunistic infections and the body's response raise energy expenditures. As people infected with HIV/AIDS experience opportunistic infections, it is important to preserve energy stores and to rest during the acute and recovery stages of the illness.[19]

In addition to good nutrition and rest, exercise is a safe and effective intervention for people with HIV for the prevention of wasting.[1] In fact, even moderate exercise has been associated with lower risk of progression to AIDS or death.[18] Both aerobic and progressive resistance exercise (weight-lifting) can lead to an increase in muscle mass, which can be an important means of preventing or forestalling AIDS wasting syndrome. Aerobic exercise also can improve cardiovascular and pulmonary function and assist the flow of lymphatic fluid through the body.

In patients without opportunistic infections who have more advanced HIV disease or even AIDS, exercise (alone or with adjunctive therapy) can lead to safe and effective repletion of lean body mass. Remember three essential points in advising exercise for people with HIV and AIDS:

1. People with current or recent opportunistic infections should reduce activity levels and rest until they have recovered to prevent additional wasting.

2. Consistent and regular exercise is important. Inconsistent exercise does not provide the benefits of conditioning or lean body mass development and may stress the immune system detrimentally.[20]

3. Moderate levels of exercise provide benefit to previously sedentary people with HIV. Strenuous exercise is not necessary to improve immunologic status and body composition.[20,24]

5. What medical therapies are used to treat wasting?

As with most serious AIDS-defining conditions, the best therapy is to prevent wasting through maximal suppression of HIV with HAART and resulting immune reconstitution. In addition to HAART and specific medications for the prevention or treatment of opportunistic infections, several pharmacologic agents are aimed at various aspects of wasting. Agents to stimulate the appetite include megestrol acetate (Megace) and dronabinol (Marinol). Megace results in weight gain, but primarily through increased fat rather than muscle mass. Adverse effects include altered glucose metabolism, hypogonadism, avascular necrosis, impotence, and, after discontinuation, adrenal insufficiency. Marinol is a marijuana derivative that stimulates the appetite and is of limited value because it does not result in significant weight gain in HIV patients. Its adverse effects include neuropsychiatric symptoms and gastrointestinal intolerance.

Anabolic steroids and recombinant human growth hormone (rhGH) have been used to promote the repletion of lean body mass. Anabolic steroids, which include testosterone ethanate, nandrolone decanoate, oxandrolone, and oxymetholone, have been shown to be effective in people with AIDS wasting syndrome, especially when combined with exercise.[5] Adverse effects include liver dysfunction, virilization (development of masculine characteristics in women, such as hirsuitism and voice change), blood clotting, and mood disorders. Recombinant human growth hormone has also resulted in the successful repletion of lean tissue. Myalgia, arthralgias, edema, hyperglycemia, and carpal tunnel syndrome have been associated with the use of rhGH.

The symptomatic and underlying treatment of diarrhea is essential in the prevention and treatment of wasting. Treatment of underlying causes of diarrhea are based on the causative agent (e.g., tuberculosis, isosporiasis, cryptosporidioidosis, *Giardia* or *Salmonella* species, amoebae). HIV enteropathy may be improved with HAART. Supplementation with the amino acid L-glutamine may help to improve the health of the intestinal mucosa. Medication-associated diarrhea may be treated with acidophilus or yogurt with live cultures, calcium supplementation, high-fiber diets, fiber supplements, and certain medications, such as loperamide or lomotil.

6. What is the lipodystrophy syndrome?

The two major components of lipodystrophy syndrome are metabolic and morphologic complications. Metabolic complications include abnormalities of glucose metabolism, hyperlipidemia, lactic acidemia/acidosis, and bone disorders. Morphologic complications include lipoatrophy, lipohypertrophy, and fat maldistribution. Although these symptoms and conditions have been grouped together in the term *lipodystrophy syndrome*, the relationship among them has not been completely determined, and a standard case definition has not been developed. The table below summarizes metabolic and morphologic complications.

Lipodystrophy Syndrome

METABOLIC COMPLICATIONS	MORPHOLOGIC COMPLICATIONS
Abnormalities of glucose metabolism 　Insulin resistance 　Glucose intolerance 　Hyperglycemia 　Diabetes (rare)	Lipoatrophy (peripheral fat loss) 　Cheeks, face 　Arms 　Legs 　Buttocks
Dyslipidemia 　Elevated total cholesterol 　Elevated LDL cholesterol 　Elevated triglycerides 　Decreased HDL cholesterol	Lipohypertrophy (central or visceral fat accumulation) 　Trunk: increased abdominal girth 　　(protease paunch, Crix[ivan] belly)
Lactic acidemia /lactic acidosis	Fat maldistribution 　Dorsocervical fat pad (buffalo hump) 　Breast enlargement 　Lipomas
Bone disorders 　Osteopenia 　Osteoporosis 　Avascular necrosis	Venomegaly (prominent veins in arms and legs 　due to loss of subcutaneous fat)

7. Discuss the prevalence of morphologic and metabolic complications among people with HIV.

The prevalence is unclear, largely because of the lack of a standard case definition. Neither isolated components of lipodystrophy syndrome nor the presence of the entire spectrum is common among all patients. The epidemiologic studies conducted to date also have been flawed because of differences in patient populations and study methodology. Wide variability exists in the ways certain dysmorphic manifestations have been assessed. Some studies have asked patients to self-report symptoms such as dorsocervical fat pads or truncal obesity. Others have relied on the more objective assessments of clinicians. The lack of baseline physical characteristics in medical records and racial differences in body shape complicate the assessment of prevalence. Some of the morphologic and metabolic changes become more prevalent in the aging non–HIV-infected population and can further confound the question of prevalence. All of these factors mean that studies must compare closely matched HIV-negative subjects with HIV-positive subjects in cross-sectional observational studies. To date, large-scale longitudinal studies have not been completed.

Nevertheless, many studies have attempted to determine the scope of the problem in the course of HIV disease and HAART therapy. Multiple lipodystrophy symptoms have been estimated to occur in a very wide range of patients on PI therapy (2–84%) and in ≤ 4% of patients not taking PIs.[3] An analysis of data from the Multicenter AIDS Cohort Study (MACS) revealed that 20% of men on HAART had a combination of peripheral fat atrophy and central fat accumulation.[7] Prevalence data from the HIV Outpatient Study (HOPS) suggest that approximately 50% of all patients on HAART have at least some evidence of morphologic change.[28] Glucose metabolic disorders have been reported in 5–17% of patients in the HOPS study, whereas the Self-Ascertained Lipodystrophy Syndrome Survey (SALSA) reported hyperglycemia in 15% of males and 6% of females.[17] Variable incidence of insulin resistance has been reported based on the class of medication: 55% of patients on PIs and 27% of those on nucleoside reverse transcriptase inhibitors (NRTIs).

8. What causes lipodystrophy syndrome?

The answer to this question is being pursued by many investigators but as yet remains unclear. Many factors have been proposed to explain various components of the problem. Because of the temporal association with the widespread use of PIs and the development of HAART, the PIs were immediately suspect. However, this finding does not imply that some or all of the components of lipodystrophy syndrome did not occur in people with HIV before the advent of HAART; certainly they were not reported as frequently. On the other hand, many of the components of lipodystrophy syndrome do not occur or occur at a much lower rate in patients who are not taking HAART therapy. The role of the NRTIs has subsequently been elucidated. Patients treated with NRTI combinations that do not include PIs are more likely to have peripheral subcutaneous fat wasting. Patients taking combinations that include PIs but not NRTIs are more likely to have visceral lipohypertrophy and metabolic complications. Patients treated with both NRTI and PI combinations are much more likely to develop lipodystrophy syndrome. Therefore, the combined toxicity of the two classes probably overlaps and has an cumulative adverse effect.

Patient factors, including age, gender, ethnic and racial background, duration of HIV infection, and duration of antiretroviral therapy, also contribute to the development of lipodystrophy; therefore, the cause is likely to be multifactorial.[7]

9. What factors have been most strongly associated with lipoatrophy?

Fat depletion or lipoatrophy has been frequently associated with use of NRTIs, most strongly with stavudine (d4T, Zerit).[14,17] Lipoatrophy occurs in patients who have used NRTIs but not PIs in the past. The duration of NRTI use is an independent predictor of fat wasting in patients on NRTI or PI therapy.

Alternatively, a recent analysis of prospective longitudinal cohort data from HOPS suggests that disease factors such as low CD4+ T cell count or large decreases in CD4 count are more closely associated with the development of lipoatrophy.[28] The MACS data also suggest a relationship between peripheral fat wasting in men and HIV infection itself.[7]

10. Have other medications been associated with lipodystrophy syndrome?

Both PIs and the NRTIs may contribute in varying degrees to the morphologic complications of HAART when used in combination. In fact, combination PI and NRTI therapy involves a much higher risk for the development of lipodystrophy than either class alone.[25]

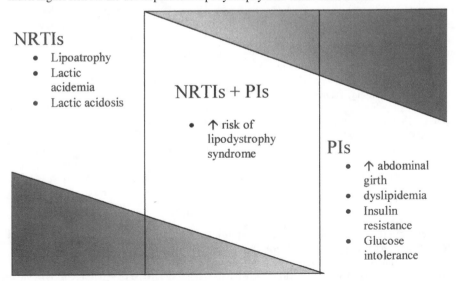

NRTIs
- Lipoatrophy
- Lactic acidemia
- Lactic acidosis

NRTIs + PIs
- ↑ risk of lipodystrophy syndrome

PIs
- ↑ abdominal girth
- dyslipidemia
- Insulin resistance
- Glucose intolerance

11. What patient factors have been associated with lipodystrophy syndrome?
Observational studies have identified several demographic factors:
• HIV infection for more than seven years
• AIDS for four years or more
• Elevated cholesterol or triglyceride levels at time of infection or initiation of HAART
• An increase of more than 2 kg/m^2 or loss of more than 1 kg/m^2 in body mass index (BMI)
• Viral load
• Prior metabolic disorders: diabetes, insulin resistance, glucose intolerance

12. When do lipodystrophy symptoms occur? Is there any difference in the onset of the various components of lipodystrophy after initiation of HAART?
Some components, particularly lipid abnormalities, can develop rather rapidly after the initiation of HAART.[16] Evidence indicates that insulin resistance develops before body composition changes and may be responsible for them. Lipoatrophy and fat redistribution are frequently not noted until after 18–24 months of therapy.[25] Data from the MACS showed an increase in lipodystrophy symptoms up to 24 months after initiation of HAART therapy; this increase leveled and did not worsen for up to another 24 months on therapy.[7] Prevalence estimates for elevated lipids in people taking PI and NRTI combinations range from 10% to 30%, and insulin resistance in the same group ranges from 10% to 20%.

13. Are there gender differences in morphologic manifestations?
Gender differences have been suggested by SALSA. Although both genders were at risk for lactic acidosis, the relative risk was higher in women. Women were also more likely to have increased abdominal fat accumulation, increased breast size, and insulin abnormalities. Men were more likely to have peripheral fat atrophy and dyslipidemia.[17] In this study the prevalence of metabolic and morphologic changes was 116 per 1000 patient years in women and 29 per 1000 patient years on therapy in men.

14. What are the clinical consequences of lipodystrophy complications?
Facial atrophy, truncal and dorsocervical fat accumulation, thin extremities, increased abdominal girth, and increased breast size are often uncomfortable and frequently quite obvious. Any of these symptoms may adversely affect self-esteem and willingness to continue HAART. Patients who observe these conditions in family members or friends may be less willing to initiate certain antiretroviral medications. Decreased adherence can lead to viral resistance and may result in future difficulty in controlling viral replication and disease progression. These outwardly visible stigmata of HIV/AIDS can cause perceived or actual problems, including discrimination and social discomfort as well as a constant reminder of the illness, its disability, and potential mortality.
Clinical symptoms directly related to the body dysmorphic features of lipodystrophy have been noted. The dorsocervical fat pad has been associated with neck pain, posture problems, and difficulty sleeping. Truncal obesity can make it difficult to breathe, can cause umbilical hernias, and can result in gastroesophageal reflux disease (GERD). Breast enlargement has been associated with pain. Most serious of all complications is the onset of the metabolic syndrome, the triad of hypertension, insulin resistance, and dyslipidemia that has been strongly associated with cardiovascular disease. Dyslipidemia, truncal obesity, and abnormalities in glucose metabolism may increase the risk of atherogenesis. These and other patient risk factors (e.g., age, gender, smoking, family history) raise the possibility of increased cardiovascular disease risk. Finally, elevated triglyceride levels (> 1000 mg/dl) are also associated with increased risk for acute pancreatitis.

15. Are patients with metabolic and morphologic conditions associated with HIV and HAART at increased risk for cardiovascular disease?
The similarity of many components of the metabolic and morphologic complications with known cardiovascular risk factors, particularly the metabolic syndrome or syndrome X, is obvious

and appropriately raises the question of increased risk for cardiovascular disease. Although the incidence of myocardial infarction seems to be increased in people infected with HIV, current data about the contribution of PIs to that risk are conflicting. The association of PIs with surrogate markers for cardiovascular disease is somewhat less ambiguous. An increased incidence of carotid atherosclerotic plaque has been demonstrated in people taking PIs.[13] The incidence of endothelial dysfunction, a risk factor for progression to cardiovascular events, has been shown to increase with use of PIs.[22]

16. What screening is considered appropriate for metabolic and morphologic complications of HAART?

Screening Tests for Metabolic and Morphologic Complications

COMPLICATION	SCREENING TEST
Insulin resistance Hyperglycemia Diabetes mellitus	Fasting blood glucose
Hypercholesterolemia Hypertriglyceridemia	Fasting lipid profile* Screening for other risk factors (NCEP ATP III guidelines)
Hyperlactatemia	Screening of asymptomatic patients not recommended
Osteopenia	Screening not recommended
Avascular necrosis	Screening not recommended
Morphologic changes	Self-reported and examiner-reported body habitus changes Standardized anthropometric measurements Bioelectrical impedance analysis Anthropometric measurement Measurement of size of dorsocervical fat pad Measurement of abdominal girth Hip-to-waist ratio

NCEP ATP = National Cholesterol Education Program Adult Treatment Panel.
* LDL-C measurements are not reliable when triglyceride levels exceed 400 mg/dl.

17. Discuss appropriate cardiovascular intervention strategies for HIV-positive people.
The first intervention is the assessment of coronary risk factors and their severity. The more severe a risk factor is, the greater the risk of cardiovascular events. Likewise, risk increases with a greater number of risk factors. The Framingham Risk Assessment, developed to determine the 10-year risk of cardiovascular events, is used to determine the appropriate level of intervention. Principles for the management of cardiovascular risk in people living with HIV are consistent with the guidelines published by the National Cholesterol Education Program Adult Treatment Panel III. However, a caveat pertains to the use of these tools. Most people with HIV are relatively young from the standpoint of cardiovascular disease, and they are living much longer in the HAART era. For these reasons, the 10-year risk assessment based on the Framingham Heart Study may not be aggressive enough for people with HIV disease. On the other hand, adherence to dietary and lifestyle modification changes are difficult enough for most members of the general population, and these lifestyle changes, added to the numerous challenges of living with and managing HIV disease, may be daunting for many patients. As in all health states, modifiable lifestyle changes are to be advised and encouraged. Smoking cessation, blood pressure control, proper diet, and exercise are essential factors in maintaining cardiovascular health in people with HIV just as in the general population.

18. Do metabolic and morphologic complications improve after the patient switches from one antiretroviral therapeutic agent or combination to another?
Better glucose metabolic parameters have been shown when patients switch from a PI to nevirapine or efavirenz in the presence of hyperglycemia, insulin resistance, and glucose intolerance.

Likewise, switching from a PI to abacavir has led to improvement in insulin tolerance and reduction in blood glucose levels. Changing from PIs to NNRTIs has had positive results in lowering cholesterol and triglyceride levels. Treatment interruption or switching agents has not resulted in significant improvement in morphologic disorders.

19. What medications are most likely to cause disorders of glucose metabolism?

PIs have direct effects on glucose metabolism[26] and are responsible for insulin resistance and impaired glucose tolerance, changes that may be precursors to later changes in body composition. The mechanism of insulin resistance is related to a number of factors, including peripheral fat atrophy, truncal obesity, increased hepatic gluconeogenesis, and the inhibition of insulin-degrading enzymes by PIs.

20. What treatments are appropriate for glucose metabolism problems?

As with frank diabetes and other glucose metabolism disorders, diet, exercise, and weight loss are the cornerstones of treatment. Pharmacologic treatment is appropriate for cases that do not respond to lifestyle modification. Oral hypoglycemic agents have been effective in helping to control glucose metabolic complications of HAART. Metformin has also been associated with weight loss, decreased blood pressure, decreased visceral adiposity, and decreased triglyceride levels. Of the thiazolidinedione class, pioglitazone has also been an effective treatment of insulin resistance, whereas rosiglitazone has shown equivocal efficacy.

21. What factors have been associated with dyslipidemia?

Lipid abnormalities were seen in HIV-infected persons before the HAART era. They were manifested primarily as low cholesterol levels and high triglyceride levels. These lipid abnormalities are believed to result from wasting and increased cytokine levels in chronic HIV infection.

After the introduction of HAART, lipid abnormalities have been clearly associated with PI therapy. Lipid elevations are common within the first few months of PI use. Among the PIs, ritonavir (Norvir) has been found to cause the greatest elevation of total cholesterol and triglyceride levels. The lipid-elevating effects of ritonavir are dose-dependent and occur with increased frequency and severity at higher dosages. Within the NRTI class, efavirenz (Sustiva) is responsible for more lipid abnormalities than other members of the class. For both PIs and NRTIs, the mechanism responsible for increased lipid levels is increased hepatic lipid production.[25]

22. Discuss treatments for dyslipidemia.

Pharmacologic interventions are used to treat lipid abnormalities in addition to NCEP ATP III assessments, interventions, and lifestyle modification. The choice of appropriate agents is determined by the specific lipid abnormality of each patient. The most frequently used medication classes are the statins and fibrates. Gemfibrozil is well tolerated and has modest effects on reduction of triglyceride levels in patients taking PIs. Pravastatin, combined with the reduction of dietary sources of fat and cholesterol, has been effective in reducing cholesterol by approximately 20%. Atorvastatin has also been used in low doses with good effect for the reduction of total and LDL cholesterol.

Other HMG CoA reductase inhibitors (especially simvastatin) should not be used with PIs because CYP 450 inhibition of statin metabolism by PIs may result in very high serum levels and an increased frequency of adverse effects. Atorvastatin should be used in lower doses with frequent monitoring. In addition, liver function tests should be monitored for the development of inflammation. Modest, short-term reductions in cholesterol and LDL have also been seen with the use of L-carnitine, 1000 mg twice daily. The table on the following page summarizes appropriate pharmacologic choices for HIV- or HAART-associated dyslipidemia.

Pharmacotherapeutic Choices for Dyslipidemia in HIV

LIPID ABNORMALITY	FIRST CHOICE	SECOND CHOICE	COMMENTS
Increased LDL-C	Statin	Fibrate	Use atorvastatin or pravastatin
Increased LDL-C and triglycerides	Fibrate or statin	May need to combine two	Monitor LFTs and CPK
Increased triglycerides	Fibrate	Statin	May need additional agents
Refractory dyslipidemias			Refer to endocrinologist for management

LDL-C = low-density lipoprotein cholesterol, LFTs = liver function tests, CPK = creatine phosphokinase.

23. What factors have been associated with osteopenia?

Although in vitro and animal model data suggest that PIs may be responsible for bone mineral resorption, the limited clinical data suggest that osteopenia may be more common in untreated HIV-positive people.[15] Other factors associated with osteoporosis and osteopenia were low calcium intake, wasting, weight loss, use of corticosteroids, and cigarette smoking. The only HAART-related factor associated with osteopenia was duration of therapy, possibly a surrogate marker for severity of HIV disease or other factors. Currently no HIV-specific guidelines have been developed for the management of osteopenia or osteoporosis. Standard guidelines for the general population should be applied as appropriate. Modifiable lifestyle factors, such as smoking cessation, resistance exercise, and adequate nutritional and calcium intake, should be stressed. In the setting of HIV-related risks for decreased bone mineral density, calcium supplements may be dually important for the management of patients with diarrhea.

24. What are lactacidemia and lactic acidosis?

Lactacidemia and lactic acidosis are the clinical spectrum of excessive lactic acid in the blood. Lactacidemia may be physiologic; the presence of elevated lactic acid is responsible for sore muscles after strenuous anaerobic exercise. In HIV, lactate is elevated because of the toxic effects of some antiretroviral medications on mitochondrial deoxyribonucleic acid (mtDNA).

25. Which medications cause lactacidemia and lactic acidosis?

The NRTIs are most frequently associated with increased serum lactacid levels, and all medications in the class have the potential for causing lactacidemia.[4,7,27] The incidence based on case reports has been estimated at 1.3 cases per 1000 person-years of NRTI treatment. In vitro studies have shown the greatest increases in lactic acid levels with zalcitabine, followed by stavudine, didanosine, tenofovir, zidovudine, abacavir, and lamivudine. Clinically the highest risk for lactacidemia comes with the use of stavudine (d4T, Zerit) or with combinations of NRTIs. The highest toxicity has been associated with d4T in combination with ddI, followed by abacavir, lamivudine, and zidovudine in combination with lamivudine. Triple nucleoside combinations have higher risk for elevated lactacidemia than single nucleosides, but they are not associated with higher risk than dual combinations of NRTIs. This toxicity has also been associated with longer duration of use of NRTIs. Other factors associated with risk for lactacidemia and lactic acidosis are female gender, obesity, coinfection with hepatitis B or hepatitis C virus, advanced AIDS, and pancreatitis. These effects are the result of NRTI toxicity on mitochondria and resolve with the discontinuation of the medication.

26. What is the mechanism of hyperlactacidemia caused by NRTIs?

Mitochondria possess their own DNA (mtDNA) and are capable of independent replication within cells in response to metabolic demands. NRTIs are believed to inhibit the mitochondrial enzyme, DNA polymerase-gamma, which is similar in form and function to HIV's own reverse transcriptase enzyme. MtDNA is responsible for the production of new mtDNA, and when it is inhibited, the production of more mitochondria is subsequently inhibited.

The process of glycolysis catabolizes glucose or glycogen, resulting in the production of pyruvate. Mitochondria continue the metabolism of pyruvate through the enzymatic reactions of oxidative phosphorylation. Without adequate amounts of mitochondria (or oxygen), pyruvate is not completely catabolized and the glycolytic byproduct lactate is produced.

27. Discuss the signs and symptoms of lactacidemia and lactic acidosis.

Lactacidemia may be asymptomatic. Symptoms generally rise with increasing hyperlactacidemia; however, they may be vague and nonspecific. Symptoms of hyperlactacidemia includes nausea, vomiting, abdominal pain, weight loss, malaise, myalgia, tachypnea, and dyspnea. Clinical findings may include decreased arterial pH, increased lactic acid levels, elevated alanine aminotransferase (ALT) levels, increased anion gap, hepatic steatosis (fatty degeneration of the liver), and pancreatitis. Bicarbonate levels may be decreased but are frequently within normal limits. Oxygen saturation levels may drop with exertion, a finding that is consistent with *Pneumocystis carinii* pneumonia. Untreated lactic acidosis has been fatal in more than 50% of reported cases.

In addition, 25 cases of hyperlactacidemia-associated ascending neuromuscular weakness, a condition similar to Guillain-Barré syndrome, have been reported. This condition has been seen among both naive and NRTI-experienced patients. Average exposure to NRTIs was 10 months, and most patients had symptoms of lactacidemia before the onset of ascending neuromuscular weakness. The most common medication associated with this condition was stavudine (d4T).

28. How is lactic acidosis treated?

Monitoring serum lactic acid levels for patients on NRTI therapy has not proved to be an effective screening tool for lactic acidosis in asymptomatic patients. Mild lactic acid elevations are not uncommon in asymptomatic patients and usually do not progress to lactic acidosis. Low-level hyperlactacidemia is not predictive of lactic acidosis. However, in symptomatic patients taking NRTIs, lactic acidosis must be considered because of the possible dire consequences of missing the diagnosis. Proper handling of serum specimens for lactic acid levels is important. Lactic acid levels may be taken from venous or arterial blood. Serum specimens for lactic acid levels should be taken without a tourniquet, if possible, and should always be the first tube drawn to ensure accurate results. Specimens should be kept cool for transport to the laboratory.

The first step in treating lactic acidosis is to discontinue all NRTIs. This step usually requires an interruption of the patient's entire HAART regimen for a certain period. Several nutritional supplements have frequently been used to treat and sometimes prevent NRTI-related mitochondrial toxicity, including L-carnitine (Carnitor) or acety-carnitine, ubiquinone (co-enzyme Q10), vitamin B_2 (riboflavin), and vitamin B_6 (pyridoxine). For lactate levels > 5 mmol/L, hospitalization is required for monitoring, IV fluids, and respiratory support. After recovery, rechallenge with NRTIs (other than stavudine) has not been associated with recurrence of lactic acidosis within 6 months.[10] The table below summarizes the management of lactacidemia and lactic acidosis.

Management of Lactadicemia and Lactic Acidosis

LACTATE LEVEL (MMOL/L)/ CLASSIFICATION	SYMPTOMS	RESPONSE
> 10 Lactic acidosis	±	Hospitalize Discontinue NRTIs
5–10 Serious hyperlactacidemia	+ +	Hospitalize Exclude other cause Discontinue NRTIs
5–10 Serious hyperlactacidemia	–	Outpatient: Exclude other cause Rule out lab error Observe

Table continued on following page

Management of Lactadicemia and Lactic Acidosis (Continued)

LACTATE LEVEL (MMOL/L)/ CLASSIFICATION	SYMPTOMS	RESPONSE
2–5 Mild hyperlactacidemia	+	Exclude other cause Consider discontinuing NRTIs
2–5 Mild hyperlactacidemia	–	Exclude other cause Observe
< 2 Normal lactate level	+	Work up symptoms Other cause for symptoms likely Observe
< 2 Normal lactate level	–	Continue therapy

BIBLIOGRAPHY

1. Arey BD, Beal MW: The role of exercise in the prevention and treatment of wasting in acquired immune deficiency syndrome. J Assoc Nurses AIDS Care 13(1):29–49, 2002 .
2. Carr A, Cooper DA: Lipodystrophy associated with an HIV-protease inhibitor. N Engl J Med 339:1296, 1998.
3. Carr A, Samaras K, Thorisdottir A, et al: Diagnosis, prediction, and natural course of HIV-1 protease-inhibitor-associated lipodystrophy, hyperlipidaemia, and diabetes mellitus: Acohort study. Lancet, 353:2093–2099, 1999.
4. Cote HCF, Brumme ZL, Craib KJP, et al: Changes in mitochondrial DNA as a marker of nucleoside toxicity in HIV-infected patients. N Engl J Med 346:811–820, 2002.
5. Fairfield W, Treat M, Rosenthal DI, et al: Effects of testosterone and exercise on muscle leanness in eugonadal men with AIDS wasting. J Appl Physiol 90:2166–2171, 2001.
6. John M, Nolan D, Mallal S: Antiretroviral therapy and the lipodystrophy syndrome. Antiviral Ther 6:9–20, 2001.
7. Kingsley L, Smitt E, Riddler S, Li R, et al: Prevalence of lipodystrophy and metabolic abnormalities in the multicenter AIDS cohort study (MACS) [abstract 538]. Presented at the 8th Conference on Retroviruses and Opportunistic Infections, Chicago, February 5–8, 2001.
8. Koch J: The role of body composition measurements in wasting syndromes. Semin Oncol 25 (2 Suppl 6):12–19, 1998.
9. Kotler DP, Tierney AR, Wang J, Pierson RN: Magnitude of body-cell mass depletion and the timing of death from wasting in AIDS. Am J Clin Nutr 50:444–447, 1989.
10. Lonergan JT, Havlir D, Barber E, Mathews WC: Incidence and outcome of hyperlactatemia associated with clinical manifestations in HIV-infected adults receiving NRTI-containing regimens [abstract 624]. Presented at the 8th Conference on Retroviruses and Opportunistic Infections, Chicago, February 4–8, 2001.
11. Macallan DC, Noble CB, Baldwin C, et al: Prospective analysis of patterns of weight change in stage IV human immunodeficiency virus infection. Am J Clin Nutr 58:417–424, 1997.
12. Macallan DC, Noble CB, Baldwin C, et al: Energy expenditure and wasting in human immunodeficiency virus infection. N Engl J Med 333(2):83–88, 1995.
13. Maggi P, Serio G, Epifani G, et al: Premature lesion of the carotid vessels in HIV-1-infected patients treated with protease inhibitors. AIDS 14:F123–F128, 2000.
14. Mallal SA, John M, Moore CB, James IR, McKinnon EJ: Contribution of nucleoside analogue reverse transcriptase inhibitors to subcutaneous fat wasting in patients with HIV infection. AIDS 14:1309–1316, 2000.
15. Mondy K, Lassa-Claxton S, Hoffmann M, Yarasheski K, Powderly W, Tebas P: Longitudinal evolution of bone mineral density (BMD) and bone markers in HIV-infected individuals. Program and abstract (718) presentation at the 9th Conference on Retroviruses and Opportunistic Infections Seattle, WA, February 24–28, 2002.
16. Mulligan K, Grunfeld C, Tai VW, et al: Hyperlipidemia and insulin resistance are induced by protease inhibitors independent of changes in body composition in patients with HIV infection. J Acq Immune Defic Syndr 23:35–43, 2000.
17. Muurahainen N, Glesby M, et al: Different factors are associated with lipohypertrophy and lipoatrophy in HIV patients with fat maldistribution. AIDS 14(Suppl):S59–S60, 2000.
18. Mustafa T, Sy FS, Macera CA, et al: Association between exercise and HIV disease progression in a cohort of homosexual men. Ann Epidemiol 9(2):127–131, 1999.

19. Paton NIJ, Elia M, Jebb SA, et al: Total energy expenditure and physical activity measured with the bicarbonate-urea method in patients with human immunodeficiency virus infection. Clin Sci 91:241–245, 1996.
20. Perna FM, LaPierriere A, Klimas N, et al: Cardiopulmonary and CD4 cell changes in response to exercise training in early symptomatic HIV infection. Med Sci Sports Exerc 31(7):973–979, 1999.
21. Serrvadda D, Mugerwam RD, Sewankambo NK, et al: Slim disease: A new disease in Uganda and its association with HTLV-III infection. Lancet 284:849–852, 1985.
22. Stein JH, Klein MA, Bellehumeur JL, et al: Use of human immunodeficiency virus-1 protease inhibitors is associated with atherogenic lipoprotein changes and endothelial dysfunction. Circulation 104:257–262, 2001.
23. Suttmann U, Ockenga J, Selberg O, et al: Incidence and prognostic value of malnutrition and wasting in human immunodeficiency virus-infected outpatients. J Acq Immune Defic Syndr Hum Retrovirol 8:239–246, 1995.
24. Terry L, Sprinz E, Ribiero JP: Moderate and high-intensity exercise training in HIV-1 seropositive individuals: A randomized trial. Int J Sports Med 20(2):142–146, 1999.
25. Van der Valk M, Gislof EH, Reiss P, et al, on behalf of the Prometheus Study group: Increased risk of lipodystrophy when nucleoside analogue reverse transcriptase inhibitors are included with protease inhibitors in the treatment of HIV-1 infection. AIDS 15:847–855, 2001.
26. Walli R, Herfort O, Michl GM, et al: Treatment with protease inhibitors associated with peripheral insulin resistance and impaired oral glucose tolerance in HIV-1-infected patients. AIDS 12:F167–F173, 1998.
27. White AJ: Mitochondrial toxicity and HIV therapy. Sex Transm Infect 77:158-173, 2001.
28. Ward D, Delaney K, Moorman A, et al: Description of lipodystrophy in the HIV Outpatient Study (HOPS) [abstract 1298]. In Proceedings of the 39th Interscience Conference on Antimicrobial Agents and Chemotherapy, San Francisco, September 26–29, 1999.

15. SEXUALLY TRANSMITTED DISEASES AND HIV

Deborah M. Frank, ACRN, MS, ANP-C

Sexually transmitted diseases (STDs) refer to the more than 25 infectious organisms transmitted through sexual activity and the multiple clinical syndromes that they cause.[7] Compared with other STDs, HIV is not easy to transmit. However, evidence indicates that ulcerative STDs (syphilis, chancroid, and genital herpes) increase the risk of HIV transmission up to 9-fold, whereas the discharge STDs (gonorrhea, chlamydial infection, and trichomoniasis) increase the risk of HIV transmission by 3–5 fold.[5] Screening for and treatment of people with STDs are important to reduce individual risk and to target high-risk communities.

1. **How do STDs function as cofactors for vaginal transmission of HIV infection?**
   A number of explanations account for the relationships between HIV infection and other STDs:
   • Disruption of the protective epithelial layers of skin and mucosal surfaces, leading to exposure of blood vessels
   • Elimination of normal, protective vaginal flora such as lactobacilli
   • Alteration of the acidic pH of the vagina
   [a] Inflammation with recruitment of CD4-positive target cells into the reproductive tract
   • Induction of inflammatory cells and release of cytokines or cell mediators that influence viral replication
   • Alteration of host cell surface properties so that attachment and entry of HIV are facilitated
   • Alteration of the biology of HIV infection by promiscuous viral gene products in cells co-infected with other intracellular pathogens[5]

2. **Discuss the major STD/HIV interrelationships.**
   HIV infectivity refers to the average probability of transmission of HIV to a person after exposure to an infected host. The triangle of behavioral, epidemiologic, and immunologic factors determines HIV infectivity.[4,8]
   • **Behavioral.** Both STDs and HIV can be sexually transmitted by rectal, vaginal, and oral intercourse.
   • **Epidemiologic.** Populations with high rates of STDs demonstrate disproportionately high rates of sexually transmitted HIV, particularly among women.
   • **Immunologic.** The presence of STDs causes changes in mucosal immunity that facilitate HIV acquisition and transmission.[4]

3. **What factors determine whether an STD or HIV will be transmitted through sexual exposure?**
   Infectivity depends on three main factors that can also be called the individual determinants of infectivity:
   • Viral dose (V)
   • Blood/mucous membrane exposure (E)
   • Host factors/resistance (R)
   The formula for determining infectivity is as follows:

$$\frac{V \times E}{R}$$

4. What factors influence viral dose or virulence?

Sexual practice affects which body fluid is present. Blood, semen, and cervicovaginal fluids are known to contain high amounts of HIV and have resulted in documented sexual transmission of HIV.[3] In women, the glandular epithelium harbors HIV in the zone of transformation between the columnar cells of the cervix, yielding HIV DNA more readily than swabs taken from the vagina (33% vs. 17%). HIV is detectable in seminal cells and seminal plasma in men. Although sperm cells do not express CD4 receptors and are unlikely to be a major source of infection, HIV DNA has been detected in some sperm cells.[8] HIV viral load in the blood is an indicator of the amount of virus in the semen or cervicovaginal fluids at any given time.

Clinical course of the disease of the infected partner. The stages of HIV disease are an important consideration in determining organism dose. As the concentration of HIV increases in the blood and probably in the genital tract, host infectiousness is also likely to increase. The period between exposure to HIV and the appearance of HIV antibodies, when primary infection occurs, has been implicated in increased infectiousness.

Antiretroviral treatment that significantly lowers the circulating copies of virus in an infected partner who adheres to therapy can significantly affect viral dose. Some studies have demonstrated decreased concentrations of seminal HIV in men taking antiretroviral therapy. Ongoing studies are attempting to determine whether antiretroviral therapy has an affect on detection of HIV in cervicovaginal specimens. A 50% reduction in sexual transmission of HIV has been reported with use of effective antiretroviral therapy.[8]

5. What factors influence exposure to HIV?

Duration and type of sexual exposure. The longer the duration of exposure for a given sexual experience, the greater the infectivity. This factor depends on the length of viability of an organism on mucous membrane surfaces and its capability for causing infection after sexual contact. For example, HIV/STD organisms ejaculated into the vagina or rectum can remain viable for up to 72 hours. Because no significant amounts of cervicovaginal or rectal fluids are introduced into the insertive partner's urethra, the urethra is exposed only during the sexual act. The abundance of Langerhans cells in the foreskin or the role of the foreskin in providing a reservoir for fluids may contribute to these findings. The prevalence of HIV infection is 1.7–8.2 times as high in men with foreskins as in men who are circumcised, and the incidence of infection is 8 times as high.[8]

Number of sexual exposures

Chance that the sexual partner is infected

6. What factors influence resistance?

Cellular immune response or mucosal immunity is recognized as the most critical factor in determining the risk of sexual transmission of HIV. Host susceptibility depends on viral entry into the cells through CD4 and chemokine surface receptors. For infection to occur, specific proteins on the envelope of HIV virus must bind to the CD4 receptors, allowing the virus to enter the cell membrane and then the nucleus of the cell, where it multiplies.

The **presence of an STD** is strongly associated with susceptibility to HIV. Ulcerations are formed when the submucosal layer of the mucous membrane is exposed through erosion of squamous or columnar epithelial cells. An inflammatory cellular immune response mobilizes T4 lymphocytes and monocyte/macrophage cells (HIV target cells) to the surfaces of the mucous membranes. The most prevalent strains of HIV in the United States are type B. Because of positive tropism for these HIV target cells, infection occurs on the surface of the mucous membranes. Although lymphocytes and macrophages are normally present in the tissues and secretions of the male and female genital tract and in the rectal mucosa of homosexual men, these HIV target cells increase in the setting of genital tract inflammation such as that associated with STDs.[9] When these monocyte/macrophage cells are infected, they act as conduits to transfer the infection into the circulation.

7. How does having an STD affect people who are HIV-seronegative?

Recruitment of HIV target cells to the surface of the mucous membranes is increased, significantly enhancing susceptibility to HIV transmission for persons with STDs. Resistance is decreased by impaired mucosal immunity, and susceptibility is increased.

$$\frac{\text{Viral dose (V)} \times \text{exposure (E)}}{\text{Decreased resistance (R)}}$$

8. How does having an STD affect persons who are HIV-seropositive?

Target cells infected with HIV are mobilized to the surface of the mucous membranes. The HIV viral load of the genital secretions is increased and the risk of HIV transmission rises. Increased viral dose increases HIV communicability and infectiousness.

$$\frac{\text{Increased viral dose (V)} \times \text{exposure (E)}}{\text{Resistance (R)}}$$

9. What are some of the specific complexities encountered in STD management of people with HIV infection?

Urethritis, pelvic inflammatory disease, genital warts, and bacterial vaginosis are among the conditions that complicate the STD management for people with HIV infection.

10. How does HIV infection affect the management of urethritis?

Urethritis or inflammation of the urethra is caused by an infection characterized by mucopurulent or purulent material and by dysuria. *Neisseria gonorrhoeae* and *Chlamydia trachomatis*, both reportable to state health departments, should be specifically diagnosed to ensure partner notification and appropriate treatment. Nongonococcal urethritis (NGU) is diagnosed if gram-negative intracellular organisms cannot be identified on Gram stains. Some of the organisms causing NGU include *C. trachomatis, Ureaplasma urealyticum, Mycoplasma genitalium, Trichomonas vaginalis*, and herpes simplex virus (HSV). Gonococcal (GC) urethritis, chlamydial urethritis, and nongonococcal, nonchlamydial urethritis may facilitate HIV transmission. HIV seminal plasma levels are increased with urethral infection compared with controls (GC > NGU). HIV seminal plasma levels in men with urethritis decrease with antibiotic treatment. Detection and treatment of urethritis may decrease the infectiousness of men with HIV infection and help to curtail the HIV epidemic.

11. Describe the effect of HIV infection on the management of pelvic inflammatory disease (PID).

PID includes a spectrum of inflammatory disorders of the upper female genital tract, including any combination of endometritis, salpingitis, tubo-ovarian abscess, and pelvic peritonitis. Although sexually transmitted organisms, especially *N. gonorrhoeae* and *C. trachomatis*, are implicated in most cases, microorganisms that can be part of the vaginal flora (anaerobes, *Gardnerella vaginalis, Haemophilus influenzae*, enteric gram-negative rods, and *Streptococcus agalactiae*) can also cause PID. *Mycoplasma hominis* and *U. urealyticum* may also be etiologic agents of PID. HIV-infected women who have PID may have more severe symptoms than HIV-negative women but seem to respond equally well to standard antibiotic regimens. Higher rates of concomitant candidal and human papillomavirus (HPV) infections and HPV-related cytologic abnormalities are seen in HIV-infected women. Hospitalization is suggested for immunosuppressed HIV-infected women with PID, and aggressive treatment with a recommended parenteral antimicrobial regimen should be initiated.

12. How does HIV infection affect the management of genital warts?

Immunosuppressed patients may not respond as well as immunocompetent people to therapy for genital warts. Recurrences after treatment are common. Squamous cell carcinoma arising in or resembling genital warts occurs more frequently in immunosuppressed people. Therefore, more frequent biopsy for confirmation of diagnosis is required.

13. Describe the effect of HIV infection on the management of bacterial vaginosis.

Bacterial vaginosis is one of the most prevalent types of vaginal infections. It is defined as replacement of the lactobacilli of the vagina by characteristic groups of bacteria, which leads to changes in the properties of the vaginal fluid. Lactobacilli are among the predominant organisms in healthy vaginal flora. Certain strains produce antimicrobial compounds such as lactic acid, hydrogen peroxide, and biosurfactants. These compounds maintain an acidic vaginal pH and prevent bacteria from adhering to the vagina and flourishing. Lactobacilli prevent colonization of pathogenic organisms, forming a barrier on the mucous membranes, neutralizing pathogens, and prohibiting their mobility. Hydrogen peroxide has been documented to have in vitro viricidal effects on HIV.[7] In addition, lactobacilli produce lactic acid, which maintains the acidic pH of the vagina. In the absence of lactobacilli, vaginal pH rises, and HIV may then more easily penetrate the vaginal epithelium.

Many factors may affect normal vaginal flora, including douching, antibiotic therapy, hormonal changes, foreign bodies (tampons, diaphragm, intrauterine device), and semen. The pH of the vagina is 3.8–4.5 (acidic), whereas the pH of semen is more alkaline (7.0–8.0). Spermicide destroys lactobacilli. HIV thrives in an alkaline environment, thus prolonging exposure time to HIV. T-lymphocytes are byproducts of bacterial vaginosis and are more receptive to HIV in an alkaline environment. Although studies suggest that bacterial vaginosis facilitates the acquisition of HIV, the role of lactobacilli is complex, and additional research is indicated to confirm and further explain its significance.[3]

14. What are the STD/HIV screening guidelines for men who have sex with men?

In New York City, the frequency of gonorrhea and infectious syphilis has shown a striking increase since 1998 in men who have sex with men. This finding represents a considerable increase in risk for transmission of HIV. "Epidemic fatigue" and "safer sex burnout" may be factors in the increasing frequency of unprotected sex, sex with anonymous partners, and related behaviors among men who have sex with men. Improved management of HIV infection and enhanced survival may also play a role.

Screening Recommendations for Men Who Have Sex with Men

Sexual history
- Sexually active with men, women, both
- Sexually active with men in the past year

All men who have had sex with other men in the preceding year
- HIV serology (if HIV-negative or not previously tested)
- Syphilis serology
- Pharyngeal culture for *Neisseria gonorrhoeae*

Men who have had receptive anal intercourse in the preceding year:
- Rectal culture for *N. gonorrhoeae* yearly
- Rectal culture for *Chlamydia trachomatis* yearly

More frequent screening (every 3–6 months) should be considered for men who acknowledge sex with anonymous male partners or multiple male partners, who use crystal methamphetamine or inhaled nitrites ("poppers"), or whose partners participate in these activities. Testing is indicated in men with symptoms of STD or HIV, regardless of when previous tests were done.

Other recommendations
- Immunization against hepatitis A and B, if unvaccinated or no prior history of infection
- Type-specific serology for herpes simplex virus (HSV). HSV type 1 and HSV type 2 are prevalent in men who sex with men. HSV infection increases the risk of acquiring and transmitting HIV, especially HSV-2. Antibody to HSV glycoprotein G accurately differentiates HSV-1 from HSV-2 antibody.

---

15. How should men who have sex with men be counseled?

Clinicians should address the following basic prevention strategies:
- Advise patients how to disclose their HIV status to all sex partners and to learn the HIV status of their partner(s).

- Encourage correct and consistent condom use for insertive and receptive anal intercourse with men and for vaginal or anal intercourse with women. The exception is when both partners in a mutually monogamous relationship of at least 3 months' duration are known to be HIV seronegative.
- Counsel patients to avoid sex with multiple or anonymous partners as well as sex in conjunction with drugs or excessive alcohol use.
- Instruct how to recognize the common symptoms of STDs and HIV infection. Advise patients to avoid sex (even with condoms) when symptoms are present.
- Recommend that patients follow the above strategies even in the presence of a low plasma HIV viral load and whether or not they are taking antiretroviral therapy. HIV can be present in semen or asymptomatic genital lesions, even when it cannot be detected in the blood.
- Encourage patients infected with HIV or other STDs to inform their sex partners and encourage them to seek evaluation and treatment.[6]

BIBLIOGRAPHY

1. Centers for Disease Control and Prevention: Guidelines for treatment of sexually transmitted diseases. MMWR 47(RR-1), 1998.
2. Centers for Disease Control and Prevention: HIV Prevention Strategic Plan through 2005. Atlanta, CDC Advisory Committee on HIV and STD Prevention, 2001.
3. Center for Health and Behavioral Training: Part II: Health Behavior Training Center's Curriculum Committee of the National Network of STD/HIV Prevention Training Center: STD/HIV Interrelationships. Rochester, NY, Center for Health and Behavioral Training, 1999.
4. Hitchcock PJ: Screening and treatment of sexually transmitted diseases: An important strategy for reducing the risk of HIV transmission. AIDS Patient Care STDs 10(2):10–15, 1996.
5. Institute of Medicine Report: The Hidden Epidemic: Confronting Sexually Transmitted Diseases. Washington, DC, Institute of Medicine, 1977.
6. New York State Department of Health Bureau of STD Control: STD/HIV Screening Guidelines for MSM. Albany, NY, New York State Department of Health Bureau of STD Control, 2001.
7. Nyirhesy P: Emerging challenges in bacterial vaginosis. Contemp Obstet Gynecol 15–28, 2000.
8. Royce RA et al: Sexual transmission of HIV. N Engl J Med 336(15):1072–1078, 1997.
9. Wasserheit JN: Epidemiological synergy. Sex Transm Dis19:61–77, 1992.

III. Vulnerable Populations

16. CHILDREN AND HIV/AIDS

Adele A. Webb, PhD, RN, ACRN, FAAN

How many times has someone told you, "Caring for children is the same as caring for adults. The equipment is just smaller"? Anyone with pediatric experience knows that this statement is not true. In fact, when caring for children with HIV/AIDS, we face many challenges that nurses caring for older populations do not have to consider. In preparing to provide such care, which often is complicated, the following questions are frequently considered.

1. How is HIV disease transmitted to infants and children?

Perinatal transmission is the most common mechanism of HIV infection in infants and children. With the advent of antiretroviral therapy during pregnancy and delivery, the number of infants infected perinatally has decreased dramatically in the United States. Perinatal transmission can occur in one of three ways: across the placenta, during labor and delivery, and from breast milk. Of the three mechanisms, most perinatal transmission occurs during labor and delivery. Thus, many sources recommend cesarean section as the preferred method of delivery. Data suggest that the rate of perinatal transmission is directly associated with the HIV level in maternal plasma. Thus, the higher the mother's viral load, the more likely the infant is to be infected.[8]

Other modes of transmission include sexual abuse, sexual assault, and sexual activity. In addition, IV drug use can lead to HIV infection in adolescents.

2. At what ages should exposed infants be tested for HIV?

Infants who have been exposed to HIV infection in utero should undergo a virologic test within the first 48 hours after birth. According to the latest research findings, nearly 40% of infected infants can be identified at that time. In addition, infants should be tested between the ages of 1 and 2 months and between the ages of 3 and 6 months. Testing at age 14 days may permit early identification of HIV infection.[6] Cord blood should not be used for HIV testing because of the potential for contamination with maternal blood. For virologic testing, a minimum of 1 cc of blood must be collected and placed into an ethylenediamine tetraacetic acid (EDTA) tube. The tube should not be overfilled. Shake the tube to prevent clotting. The specimen can be kept at room temperature.[7]

3. What are the diagnostic criteria for HIV infection in infants and children?

Diagnostic Criteria for HIV Infection in Infants and Children

CATEGORY	CRITERIA
Age < 18 mo	Is known to be HIV-positive or born to an HIV-positive mother *and* Has positive results on two separate determinations from one or more of the following HIV detection tests: • HIV culture • HIV DNA polymerase chain reaction • HIV antigen *or* Meets criteria for AIDS diagnosis based on the 1987 AIDS surveillance case definition

Table continued on following page

Diagnostic Criteria for HIV Infection in Infants and Children (Continued)

CATEGORY	CRITERIA
Age ≥ 18 mo	Is born to an HIV-positive mother or infected by blood, blood products, or other known modes of transmission *and* Is HIV antibody-positive by repeated reactive enzyme immunoassay (EIA) and confirmatory test (e.g., Western Blot) *or* Meets any of the criteria for the child < 18 mo of age
Perinatally exposed child who does not meet above criteria	Is HIV-seropositive by EIA and confirmation tests performed at < 18 mo of age *or* Has unknown antibody status but born to mother known to be infected with HIV
Seroreverter (child born to HIV-positive mother)	Has been documented as HIV-antibody negative *and* Has had no other laboratory evidence of infection *and* Has not had an AIDS-defining condition[5]

4. What are the common symptoms of HIV infection in infants and children?

Children with HIV disease suffer from many of the same childhood infections as other children, but they seem to acquire these infections with increased frequency.[11] Conditions such as ear infections, pneumonia, gastroenteritis, fever, and diarrhea tend not only to occur more often in children with HIV disease but also to be more persistent and more severe. Less common conditions, such as enlarged lymph nodes and enlarged liver, are prevalent in children with HIV.[11]

Early clinical signs of HIV disease may be nonspecific. Often they are indicative of a systemic illness. Infants and children presenting with failure to thrive and developmental delay may be demonstrating early signs of HIV infection. The fact that many of the signs and symptoms of HIV disease are similar to the symptoms of other childhood diseases often obscures the suspicion of HIV and prolongs the diagnosis.[10]

5. When should antiretroviral therapy be initiated in infants and children?

According to the Centers for Disease Control and Prevention (CDC), the following guidelines provide optimal treatment of infants and children infected with HIV:

- Clinical symptoms associated with HIV infection
- Evidence of immune suppression, indicated by CD4 T-cell absolute number or percentage
- Age < 12 months, regardless of clinical, immunologic, or virologic status
- For asymptomatic children aged ≥ 1 year with normal immune status, two options can be considered:
  1. Initiate therapy, regardless of age or symptom status
  2. Defer treatment in situations in which the risk for clinical disease progression is low and other factors favor postponing treatment. In such cases, the health care provider should regularly monitor virologic, immunologic, and clinical status.[6]

Combination therapy is recommended with emphasis on the importance of adherence to prevent resistance.

6. What are the issues related to adherence in the treatment of HIV-infected children?

Combination antiretroviral therapy is the gold standard of treatment for HIV-infected children. Adhering to an often complex regimen is difficult for any patient, but certain issues related to HIV treatment make adherence more difficult for children.

First and foremost is the fact that children must rely on their parents for medications. Parents who work or are often away from their children have difficulty in maintaining a rigid medication schedule. In addition, if babysitters or other caregivers are not aware of the child's HIV diagnosis, parents may be hesitant to send the HIV medication for administration by the caregiver.

Some medications are not available in liquid formulations. Others are not tasty and over time become more and more difficult to administer to young children. School-aged children and adolescents may not want to take their medications at school. They are also old enough to relate the side effects that they may suffer directly to the medication. This detail alone may be sufficient cause to discontinue taking the drug. Other issues, such as guilt from the parent in the case of perinatal transmission or lack of understanding of the importance of adherence, are also paramount in the adherence dilemma.

7. How does HIV disease progress in infants and children?

Two general patterns of clinical illness are found in children with HIV disease. Rapid progressors are infants who develop serious disease quite quickly and often die during the first year of life. Most children have a much slower rate of disease progression; however, perinatally infected children generally develop symptoms by 2 years of age.[9]

Signs and symptoms most commonly found in children with HIV disease include failure to thrive, chronic diarrhea, wasting, oral thrush, and fever. Over time, destruction of the immune system leads to an increase in the number and severity of serious bacterial infections. Opportunistic infections, such as lymphoid interstitial pneumonitis, further compromise the health of the child. Common pathogens, such as respiratory syncytial virus, can result in serious illness in the HIV-infected child.[10]

8. Can opportunistic infections be prevented in infants and children?

Prophylaxis for opportunistic infections is based on CD4 counts with the exception of *Pneumocystis carinii* pneumonia (PCP) prophylaxis, which is given to all infants born to HIV-infected women at age 4–6 weeks. The following table summarizes the guidelines for antimicrobial prophylaxis in HIV-infected infants and children.[4,7,10]

Prophylaxis for Opportunistic Infections in Infants and Children

		CRITERIA FOR INITIATION	
INFECTION	DRUG/DOSE	AGE	CD4 COUNT
Mycobacterium avium complex	Clarithromycin, 7.5 mg/kg (not to exceed 500 mg) orally 2 times/day *or* Azithromycin, 20 mg/kg (not to exceed 1200 mg) orally weekly	< 1 yr 1–2 yr 2–6 yr > 6 yr	< 750 < 500 < 75 < 50
Pneumocystis carinii pneumonia	Trimethoprim ,150 mg/M²/day plus sulfamethoxazole, 750 mg/ M²/day orally in 2 divided doses 3 times per week on consecutive days	4–6 wk of life: all infants born to HIV-positive mothers (continue until 12 mo of age or confirmation of HIV seronegativity) 1–5 yr 6–12 yr	< 500 < 200
Cytomegalovirus	Ganciclovir, 30 mg/kg orally 3 times/day	CD4 < 50 *and* CMV antibody positivity	
Histoplasmosis	Itraconazole, 2–5 mg/kg orally every 12–24 hr	CD4 < 50 *and* residence in endemic areas	
Oral candidiasis	Not recommended		
Esophageal candidiasis	Not recommended		
Coccidioidomycosis	Not recommended		

9. Should immunizations be given to an HIV-infected infant or child?

In general, immunizations are safe for HIV-infected infants and children. However, these children often receive less benefit from the immunizations than HIV-negative children because of immune suppression.[10] Immunization can cause a temporary increase in HIV viral load, but this increase does not appear to have adverse consequences for the child.

Both HIV-positive and HIV-exposed children should be immunized with nonlive vaccines, according to the most recent American Academy of Pediatrics guidelines.[1] Apart from the measles, mumps, and rubella (MMR) vaccine, children with HIV infection should *not* be given live virus vaccines. Even if uninfected, children receiving oral polio vaccine pose a risk to any HIV-infected adults in the family.[12] Only HIV-positive children who are not severely immune compromised can receive the MMR. However, if exposed to the measles, even immunized HIV-positive children require imunoglobulin prophylaxis.

All HIV-positive children should be immunized with the 23-valent polysaccharide pneumococcal vaccine at 24 months of life.[5] Revaccination is recommended after 3–5 years for children ages 10 and younger and after 5 years for children older than 10 years. HIV-positive children should also be given yearly influenza vaccinations beginning at 6 months of age.[12]

10. How can we help parents cope with an HIV diagnosis in their child?

To help parents cope with caring for a child with HIV infection, a comprehensive assessment of the family is essential. It is important to know what family members understand about the diagnosis. Do they understand transmission, and are they able to prevent transmission in the home? Are they ready to acknowledge that the child is infected, or are they planning on nondisclosure? What is the health status of the parents? Is one or both infected with HIV?

Whether or not one of the parents is also infected, it is imperative to assess the family's social support system. Which people can help the family? Are they willing and able to provide day or respite care for the child? Is the family in a stable economic situation? Are parents able to provide for the child's nutrition and medication needs?

Most importantly, health care providers must remind parents that, aside from the HIV diagnosis, their child is still a child with all the needs related to healthy growth and development. Anticipatory guidance related to safety, nutrition, sleep, exercise, discipline, and health maintenance needs to be provided at every opportunity.[12]

BIBLIOGRAPHY

1. American Academy of Pediatrics Committee on Infectious Diseases and Committee on Pediatric AIDS: Measles immunization in HIV infected children. Pediatrics 103:1057–1060, 1999.
2. Butz AM, Joyner M, Friedman DG, Hutton N: Primary care for children with human immunodeficiency virus infection. J Pediatr Health Care 12(1):10–19, 1998.
3. Centers for Disease Control and Prevention: Revised classification system of human immunodeficiency virus infection in children less than 13 years of age. MMWR 43(RR-12):3, 1994.
4. Centers for Disease Control and Prevention: 1995 Revised guidelines for prophylaxis against *Pneumocystis carinii* pneumonia for children with or perinatally exposed to human immunodeficiency virus infection. MMWR 44(RR-4):1, 1995.
5. Centers for Disease Control and Prevention: 1997 USPHS/IDSA guidelines for the prevention of opportunistic infections in persons infected with human immunodeficiency virus. MMWR 46(RR-12):1–46, 1997.
6. Centers for Disease Control and Prevention: Guidelines for the Use of Antiretroviral agents in Pediatric HIV Infection. Atlanta, Centers for Disease Control and Prevention, 2001.
7. Dunn AM: Children with HIV/AIDS. In Kirton CA, et al (eds): Handbook of HIV/AIDS Nursing. St. Louis, Mosby, 2001, pp 380–420.
8. Johnson JP, et al: Natural history and serological diagnosis of infants born to human immunodeficiency virus infected women. Am J Dis Child 143:1147, 1989.
9. Mayaux MF, et al. Neonatal characteristics in rapidly progressive perinatally acquired HIV-1 disease. JAMA 275:606, 1996.
10. Moss W, Persaud D: Human immunodeficiency virus Infection and acquired immunodeficiency syndrome. In Hoekelman RA, et al (eds): Primary Pediatric Care, 4th ed. St. Louis, Mosby, 2002, pp 1543–1549.
11. Pizzo PA, Wilfert CM (eds.): Pediatric AIDS: The Challenge of HIV Infection in Infants, Children, and Adolescents, 3rd ed.. Baltimore, Williams & Wilkins, 1998.
12. Raszka WV: Pediatric human immunodeficiency type 1 infection. In Green-Hernandez C, Singleton J, and Aronzon DZ (eds): Primary Care Pediatrics. Philadelphia, J.B. Lippincott, 2001, pp 843–861.

17. ADOLESCENTS AND HIV/AIDS

Richard S. Ferri, PhD, ANP, ACRN, FAAN

Adolescents are generally overlooked in the HIV/AIDS pandemic. However, one in five newly diagnosed cases of HIV infection is in the 20–29 age group. It is believed that many of these young adults were infected as teenagers. In addition, the World Health Organization (WHO) estimates that half of the 14 million people living with HIV disease worldwide were infected between the ages of 15 and 24. Adolescents are a highly vulnerable cohort that needs special consideration for prevention and treatment.

1. What developmental characteristics place adolescents at increased risk for acquiring HIV infection?

Adolescence is a time of experimentation with various roles and risk-taking behaviors. Most teenagers do not have the life experience and maturity of their adult counterparts. They have a tendency to live in the "here and now" without focusing on potential consequences of their behaviors. This characteristic is seen not only in sexual activity but also in the rate of cigarette smoking, high-speed driving, and binge drinking. Negative peer pressure may also influence behaviors.

The phenomenon of "teenage bravado" has been described as a sense of invulnerability that increases risk-taking behaviors. Because most adolescents have not seen someone with HIV infection live and die with the disease, they feel that "it happens to other (older) people."

2. Are all adolescents alike?

Certainly not. Adolescents, like adults, have many different qualities that make up their being, such as race, religion, sexuality, and ethnicity. These important factors need to be considered in developing any educational or preventive program aimed at teens. In short, know your audience.

3. Discuss the issues related to gay, lesbian, bisexual, and questioning teenagers.

Gay, lesbian, bisexual, and questioning teenagers have additional needs that are frequently overlooked. They have to deal with the issues surrounding identity formation ("coming out") and the associated social implications. They also may be fearful of family and peer rejection. Many teenagers who come out are rejected and find themselves homeless. This situation may lead to economically coerced sexual behavior ("survival sex") or recreational sexual activity ("comfort sex").

It is estimated that the gay questioning or identifying teenager will have his first sexual experience with a male seven years his senior. The teenager may be fearful of approaching a peer or simply unaware of where to socialize with other gay teenagers. This problem typically can be seen in the gay teenager's feeling that "I'm the only one like this in the world." Sexual activity with an experienced adult increases the likelihood of acquiring a sexually transmitted infection, including HIV.

Finally, a very sad but real factor that affects the gay teenager and the rate of HIV infection is the treatment advances that are so helpful to infected patients. Many teenagers simply do not see HIV disease as a frightening issue any more and mistakenly believe that, if they become infected, all they have to do is "take pills." They are not aware of the profound side effects, the daunting need for adherence, and the impact on daily functioning. Some gay teenagers simply see HIV disease as "a rite of passage."

4. How does alcohol and substance abuse affect teenagers in the age of HIV/AIDS?

Any substance that reduces social inhibitions can increase the likelihood of acquiring HIV infection. Adolescents often experiment with alcohol and drug use. Several national high school surveys of school-based use of alcohol and substances have produced alarming results, such as the finding that 17.9% of high school students claim to drink at least monthly and 9.9% report weekly alcohol consumption.

As illicit drug prices decrease on the street, use increases in the adolescent community. Crack cocaine is readily available and financially feasible for many teenagers. Crack is highly addictive and acts as a sexual stimulant.

In addition, the use of mind-altering substances, especially in the adolescent age group, decreases compliance with condom use. Nearly 25% of adolescents report failure to use a condom after drug use.

5. Discuss the epidemiology of HIV infection in adolescents.

Although the overall rate of HIV infection is decreasing in the United States, there is an increase in the adolescent community. The true rate of HIV infection is believed to be greatly underreported in the adolescent community because of the lack of adolescent-sensitive HIV antibody testing programs, fear of diagnosis, and teenagers' failure to perceive the need for testing.

In addition, the current Centers for Disease Control and Prevention (CDC) age grouping is far too restrictive and does not reflect the true scope of the pandemic. For example, the adolescent age grouping for CDC-defined AIDS is ages 13–19 years. However, the vast majority of teenagers with HIV disease do not develop AIDS by the age of 19, thereby providing a false impression of low infection rates.

When back calculation of the HIV statics between 1989 and 1992 was performed, one out of every four persons in the United Stated infected with HIV was under the age of 22.

6. How is primary prevention of HIV infection different for the adolescent community?

Primary prevention interventions should be multidimensional and target the specific adolescent age group. In other words, what may be appropriate for 13-year-olds may not be applicable to the 17-year-old cohort. Basic principles of adolescent primary prevention strategies include the following:

- Programs should offer multiple options for behavioral change—not just one strategy.
- Positive peer pressure is highly effective. Adolescents have a need to conform to their peer group.
- Skills-building workshops are necessary to help the teenagers learn negotiation skills and resist negative peer pressure.
- Self-efficacy is critical. Adolescents who believe they can carry out a skill successfully have an increased chance of doing so.
- Cultural identity and inclusion may make the learning experience more meaningful to the teenager.
- Heterosexuality should *not* be the presumed norm of the group. Gay and bisexual roles and relationships should be explored.

7. Is "abstinence-only" education the best way to help stem HIV infection in teenagers?

In a resounding word, *no!* Abstinence-only programs presume heterosexuality and tell the teenager that sexually activity needs to "wait for marriage." Because gay and lesbian people are prohibited from marriage, this message does not apply to gay teenagers. Typically what happens is that anyone who does not see himself in the category of "getting married" tunes out the information.

In addition, several studies that examined abstinence-only programs have found some disturbing results. First, when teenagers are questioned about "waiting until marriage," they can repeat essentially everything that was said in the program. However, when the same teenagers are questioned about their sexual activity, they respond that they are *more* sexually active than teenagers who attend education programs that offer multiple options and skills. Such findings do not mean that abstinence education is not a vital component in primary HIV prevention education. It should be discussed in the context of other interventions but not as the sole skill.

8. Are the health and primary care needs different for adolescents and adults with HIV infection?

The health care needs of all people living with HIV infection are constantly evolving. HIV has never been a static disease. Clinicians should always refer to the latest treatment guidelines, which can be found at http://www.hivatis.org. This "living document" is constantly updated and serves as a good source of information.

The health care needs of adolescents may differ from those of adults, depending on when they become infected. Adolescents who are infected at a very young age as or as children will more than likely display some delays in growth and development milestones. It is also critical that their immunization status be up to date.

Parents or caregivers may need additional information and education about the effect of the routine diseases of childhood on teenagers with HIV infection. In addition, if there is "something going around the school," it may be wise to keep the teenager at home.

BIBLIOGRAPHY

1. Ferri R: The needs of special populations: Adolescents and persons with hemophilia. In Ungvarski PJ, Flaskerud JH (eds.): HIV/AIDS: A Guide to Primary Care Management. Philadelphia, W.B. Saunders, 1998.
2. Ferri R: HIV antibody testing and counseling. In Cohen FL, Durham JR (eds): The Person with HIV/AIDS: Nursing Perspectives. New York, Springer, 2000.
3. Ferri R: Differential diagnosis: Opportunistic infections in the era of highly active antiretroviral therapy. Primary Care Pract 4(1): 20–28, 2000.

Websites
AIDS Education Global Information System: http://www.aegis.com
World Health Organization: http://www.who.int

18. WOMEN AND HIV/AIDS

Rosanna F. DeMarco, PhD, RN, ACRN, and
Christine Johnsen, MS, MPH, RN, ANP

The human immunodeficiency virus (HIV) has been addressed in much of the health care community from a biomedical perspective. This approach marginalizes women. Social, cultural, and gender-specific needs of women are "silenced" because reliance on scientific solutions through immunology or virology does not examine the social and cultural contexts that render certain people more vulnerable than others.

1. Why are women considered a vulnerable population?

Women are more vulnerable than men, especially in developing countries, and women of color are particularly vulnerable—economically, socially, physically, and sexually. In all of these areas, women with HIV are most vulnerable.

2. Describe the economic vulnerability of women.

Many women depend on men for economic support. Many countries preferentially educate and employ men. Most of women's work is unpaid: child care, meal preparation, laundry, and housekeeping. Women with HIV are more likely to be impoverished, affecting their ability to stay healthy by limiting their access to food, shelter, and medical care. Options for paid employment outside of sex work are quite restricted in many societies. Women are more likely to be responsible for nursing ill family members, further affecting their economic situation. Susser and Stein[16] reported that women in South Africa stated that the best method for preventing HIV was to provide work for women.

3. How are women vulnerable in social terms?

Women often marry or have sex with older men who have had more sexual partners and who are thus more likely to be infected.[14] In sub-Saharan Africa, girls between 15 and 19 years old are 5–6 times more likely to be HIV-infected than their male peers.[3] Women often lack the right to make their own decisions about reproductive health and childbearing. Many societies do not recognize the legal rights of women in custody battles, tying women to their husbands to remain with their children. Women often are unable to negotiate safer sex practices. Women addicts are more likely to be the second or last user to share a needle and syringe and may be too intimidated to clean it in the presence of their shooting partners.[5,13] Hispanic-American and African-American women, who are most affected by HIV, have limited advocacy organizations and resources to protect their rights.

4. Discuss the physical vulnerability of women.

Women are physically more vulnerable and more likely to have experienced violence in their lives for several complex reasons related to the physical power of men over women, social circumstances, and cultural beliefs. Women are subject to trafficking, forced prostitution, rape (including marital rape), and incest. Women and children are most vulnerable to the consequences of displacement and forced migration. Women and girls are especially vulnerable to sexual violence during war, civil conflict, and refugee life. Worldwide, between 85 and 114 million girls and women have been "circumcised." Female genital mutilation (FGM) has severe health consequences, including facilitating the transmission of HIV. Even though FGM is practiced mostly in Islamic countries, it is not an exclusively Islamic practice. FGM is a cross-cultural and cross-religious ritual. In Africa and the Middle East it is performed by Muslims, Coptic Christians, members of various indigenous groups, Protestants, and Catholics, to name a few. FGM has often

125

been called female circumcision and compared with male circumcision. However, such comparison is often misleading. Both practices include the removal of well-functioning parts of the genitalia and are quite unnecessary. Both rituals also serve to perpetuate customs that seek to regulate and keep control over the individual's body and sexuality However, FGM is far more drastic and damaging than male circumcision. To put this behavior in perspective, a clitoridectomy would be analogous to removal of the entire penis from a man.[1,4]

5. What are the historical and epidemiologic trends in HIV/AIDS for women?
Worldwide, women account for 47% of the 36.1 million adult HIV cases, and this rate is steadily increasing. There are two epidemics: one in industrialized countries and one in developing countries. In industrialized countries, HIV morbidity and mortality have decreased significantly as a result of highly active antiretroviral therapy (HAART). Perinatal HIV transmission has also declined dramatically. In developing countries, the lack of infrastructure and education, the high cost of medications, and the poor state of sexual and reproductive health services for women are major sources of ill health and major determinants of the spread of HIV among women.[7]

Women account for an increasing proportion of reported AIDS cases in the United States—most recently, about 24% of adult AIDS cases. Women of color account for 80% of women with AIDS compared with 61% of men with AIDS. African-American women have an AIDS rate 25 times greater than white women; Hispanics have a rate 7 times greater than Caucasians. It is estimated that 62% of HIV infections in women are acquired through heterosexual transmission and 34% through injection drug use. Other factors include other percutaneous exposure (e.g, needlesticks, transfusions) and unknown risks.[2]

Women are diagnosed later and begin treatment at a later stage than men. They have increased morbidity and mortality rates. In most studies, women have a shorter duration of infection before development of AIDS and death than men.[2]

6. How do women get and transmit the virus?
The major sources for women receiving and transmitting HIV are sexual and parenteral. The incidences of these and other sources of transmission are listed in the following table:

Estimated Risk Per Event

Sexual	
Receptive anal sex	0.1–0.3%
Receptive vaginal sex	0.1–0.3%
Insertive vaginal sex	0.1%
No published estimates of risk of oral-vaginal, oral-anal, and digital intercourse, but instances have occurred.	
Parenteral	
Transfusion after single unit of infected whole blood or clotting factors	95%
Sharing needles	0.67%
Occupational needlestick	0.4%
Perinatal	
In utero	5%
Intrapartum	20%
Breastfeeding	15%
Other factors	
Presence of other sexually transmitted diseases	Menstruation
High viral load	Lack of circumcision in male partner
Trauma during sex	Nonoxynol 9

Adapted from Anderson J (ed): A Guide to the Clinical Care of Women with HIV. Washington, DC, Health Resources and Services Administration, 2000, p. 3.

7. Discuss the connections among women, violence, and HIV.

There is a strong relationship among women, violence, and HIV.One in three women worldwide is beaten, coerced into sex, or abused in her lifetime, and a partner or ex-partner will physically assault one in five to one in three of all women in the United States during their lifetime. The current or former partner kills one-half of women murdered in the U.S. Women in many countries report that raising the issue of condom use can lead to a violent response.

The prevalence of physical and sexual abuse histories among HIV-infected women is high—in one study, 68%. Women who have been abused as children are more likely to report increased risky behaviors, including multiple sexual partners, unprotected sex, substance abuse, and the ongoing experience of violence in their lives. Early sexual abuse leads to later abuse and violence.[2]

Women who have reported both physical and sexual abuse are significantly more likely to have experienced sexually transmitted disease, evidence of their increased risk. The prevalence of domestic violence among women at risk for HIV is high; one in five HIV-infected women reported that interpersonal violence contributed to their HIV positivity.

8. Why do biomedical models of research and care create barriers for women living with HIV?

In 1976, after the Dalkon shield disaster, the Federal Drug Administration (FDA) responded to demands by women's health advocates by tightening regulations for female condom devices. The new regulations, however, made no distinction between internal devices and vaginal barrier devices. It is more difficult to obtain FDA approval of simple vaginal devices. As a result, women have less access to protective measures.

Another barrier for women—and perhaps men, if they support use of female condoms—is the cost of female condoms relative to male condoms. Vaginal condoms are three times as expensive as male condoms. Because of the difference in cost, male condoms are more readily available and accessible as "free" in clinics and harm-reduction programs.

Conventional cognitive-behavioral theories often do not work well for women. For example, improving perceived control is ineffective for safer sex practices if the real control resides with the partner. The need is to focus on community empowerment—not just individual empowerment—to give women more control over safer sex.[13]

9. What interventions may help to empower women?

To empower means to grant power. Power is the ability to act effectively, to exercise control. Empowerment gives a woman control over her situation and actions. Education is a major strategy for empowerment. The following interventions are recommended:

- **HIV education.** There is a need to educate women at an appropriate literacy level, with understandable terminology that is culturally appropriate and sensitive. Education programs targeting both men and women must incorporate ways of raising the status and value of women. The curriculum should include (1) basic HIV transmission information; (2) harm reduction education; (3) practical skills, such as negotiating safer sex; and (4) teaching women to value themselves as full and equal partners.
- **Economic independence** is crucial to enable women to make certain decisions for themselves. Women need job training, through adult education programs, on-the-job training, and vocational educational programs designed to serve women at risk. Businesses should be offered incentives to provide micro-loans to foster women's economic development.
- **Practical support** is vital to women's empowerment. Women need food, safe housing, transportation, and child care. Referrals to social service and community-based organizations can assist women in obtaining needed resources.
- **Medical services.** A change in paradigm from a male-dominated health care decision model to a collaborative approach that is gender-sensitive is imperative for empowerment of women. Interventions include (1) female-controlled methods of HIV prevention and (2) family-centered health care.

10. What are the key predictors of morbidity and mortality in women?

Characteristics of HIV-infected women differ significantly from characteristics of HIV-infected men. They differ most profoundly by socioeconomic status (SES), culture, race/ethnicity, risk behavior for HIV, social support, and caregiver responsibilities. After controlling for SES, injection drug use (IDU),and race/ethnicity, very few differences in morbidity and mortality exist between women and men with HIV infection. This does not take into consideration gynecologic or obstetric issues. It is reasonable to believe that these predictors are significant issues that define the nature of the chronic course and prevalence of illness for women.

11. What type of supports specifically address women and their families?

Friedemann[11] suggests that women living with HIV/AIDS can benefit when nurses ask them to assess their individual and family behaviors and focus support based on these self-assessments. She suggests using a framework that identifies behaviors from the point of view of four concepts:

- **Coherence** represents behaviors that sustain unity and indicates how connected a woman feels to others or her individual perceptions of her family's connection to others.
- **Maintenance** is directed at the perception of keeping stability and control over a situation. The behaviors are aimed at meeting physical, emotional, and social needs and can be compared with self-care. Examples are sleeping, eating, and working. The key indicator is behavior that resists change.
- **Change** is indicated by tension or unhappiness with a current situation that compels the person or family to test values and set new priorities in life.
- **Individuation** is an action of venturing out into the environment and applying oneself in a search for meaningful experiences.

Each of these concepts ideally creates congruence or balance as a state of wellness and health. Nurses can ask women living with HIV/AIDS to address these four behaviors first as they relate to their own self-assessment and then as they they relate to their family.

12. Give examples of key supports for women and their families.

Key supports include an exploration of the client's current perceptions of behaviors and what she would like to address in the future as goals. For example, an HIV-positive woman may live with her significant other and three children ranging in age from 3 to 16 years. At this stage, the family must deal with the chronic illness of one of its members. This goal requires them to promote coherence and maintenance behaviors. The nurse can ask what specific family goals are related to the other key concepts of change and individuation. For women and their families, this approach often takes the form of opening a conversation related to what specifically and uniquely would help them test some of their values and move in the direction of finding meaning in their lives. Perhaps being part of a support group that helps others who are addressing the disease would help them find meaning. Perhaps, individually or as a family, they can think of what they value and see if some of those values can be changed to help sustain the care needed for the woman who is chronically ill. A woman with HIV/AIDS stated that when she realized how much she put others before herself as a value in her family, she began to think about how she may redirect those efforts to pay attention to her own needs as well.[10]

13. What community resources are available for women and their families?

Community resources include HIV/AIDS formal and informal groups that are institution- or community-based. In some cases, the outreach programs include invitations for women to come to social gatherings with or without their families to enjoy interactions with health care professionals, community volunteers, and other affected women. The social gatherings offer an opportunity to share educational and support programming through fliers or word of mouth. Retreats for spiritual support, economic assistance, and programs offering advice from health care professionals related to psychosocial and physical symptoms are offered. These programs use a variety of formats that may include not only attendance at an event or program but also the use of video,

CD-ROM, and Internet media as a means for communication and connection. Lastly, many grass-root efforts harness women affected by HIV/AIDS as sources of support and education across generations in school systems or neighborhoods. Many of these groups are often defined and made up of women of a specific cultural group. These groups can reach out to other women who share common heritage and community.

14. What key variables have shown an important influence on quality of life for HIV-infected women?

Significant variables that affect quality of life are substance abuse and violence. It is important to address the issue from a gender, cultural, and social support perspective. Power inequities and the social and cultural forces that shape women's risk behaviors need exploration. Concurrent and ongoing drug treatment is the necessary first step toward assisting women in taking care of their own health. An understanding of how these risk behaviors affect women's adjustment to chronic illness is extremely important in their long-term care.

Women need to know that health care providers pay attention to the unique side effects of current antiretroviral therapies and their impact on quality of life. Information about medication side effects has largely been based on the experience of men enrolled in clinical trials. Quality of life is enhanced when women feel that their symptoms are taken seriously with appropriate follow-up.[10]

Because the majority of women living with AIDS (77%) are African-American and Hispanic-American, it is important to understand quality of life from a perspective of untangling the concepts of race, culture, and ethnicity for individual women and their families.[6] Acculturation affects how women appraise their illness and their quality of life.

Lack of adequate social support is related to increased depression, less fighting spirit, and poor adjustment to illness.[17] Addressing social support needs is significant and complex. For women who actively abuse substances, family conflict related to this behavior makes connections tenuous at best. Low SES predicts a greater need for tangible support among African-American women. Because women living with HIV/AIDS are often caregivers for others in their family, they frequently provide care in the context of poverty, although this is not always the case. For women who are poor, living with chronic illness may be less of a problem than dealing with issues associated with poverty. Thus, a cumulative effect may develop related to the stressors identified by women in their unique situations.

15. What key variables have shown an important influence on adherence?

Adherence to therapeutic regimens involves a variety of behaviors that include attending to health care appointments and taking prescribed medication. For women the qualities of the health care provider involved in their care and social supports are the most important influences for adherence. Women living with HIV/AIDS express the need for sensitivity of the health care provider, i.e., being a good listener and a compassionate presence. In many instances, if the health care provider is a woman, women with HIV/AIDS feel more open to disclosure and to listening to suggestions.[9,10] Women with HIV/AIDS feel comforted by other women, not only in social support circles but also in the health care setting. Because of the key connection between women and their families, particularly their children, provision of day care or developmentally appropriate psychological support for the family helps women be attentive to their own needs.

16. How do gender theories inform the health care providers about caring for this group of clients/patients?

Many gender theories and much feminist literature propose that women often maintain behaviors that preserve personal and professional relationships at all costs. According to DeMarco et al.,[9] women create, maintain, and sustain social relationships that are based on gender-specific norms. This framework is superimposed on women who live with HIV/AIDS. Researchers and educators have attested that the primary socialization of women is perpetuated as an ideology that creates a woman-specific world based on their unique way of "knowing."[12] Silencing is one of the formidable behaviors that can educate health care providers about women's responses at the interface of care received from the health care system and interactions with those who are significant in their personal lives.

17. Discuss the importance of silencing and depression.

Jack[15] first discussed the concept of silencing in her 1991 book, *Silencing the Self: Women and Depression*. Jack traces many issues that support the contention that depression is a complex, multifaceted illness, influenced by numerous biologic and psychosocial factors. The focus of her exploration is women's mental health, and she asserts that developmental, clinical, and psychoanalytic psychologists agree that "women's orientation to relationships is the central component of female identity and emotional activity"[15] (p. 3). However, Jack contends that, when appraised in a cultural context, this healthy capacity for intimacy and maturity has been viewed as a weakness by society, psychologists, psychological measurement tools, and, most importantly, women themselves. Female caretaking and male dominance emerge as themes. Women emulate their mothers and the female caretaking role, which forces society to develop separate distinctions based on gender differences. Daughters mature to adulthood with many aspects of the mother-child relationship still intact. Sons relinquish the closeness and form an identity separate from their maternal bond.

Jack contends that "women's vulnerability to depression does not lie in their dependence on relationships or in their depressive response to loss, but in what happens to them within their relationships . . . . Missing from most accounts of depression are the entanglements that result when intimacy occurs within a context of inequality"[15] (p. 21). The traditional theories and measures of depression have not adequately taken into account the feminine relational sense of self, gender norms, and societal and cultural inequalities. Jack[15] gained better insight into the nature of depression in women and concepts that "more adequately reflected women's emotional realities" (p. 23) by interviewing depressed women in order that they, rather than "interpreters" of their experience, would honestly represent their feelings and emotions.

18. What is the Silencing the Self Scale (STSS)?

Jack's research revealed that, in order to maintain safe, intimate relationships, women silence certain feelings, thoughts, and actions. "This self-silencing contributes to a fall in self-esteem and feelings of a 'loss of self' as a women experiences, over time, the self-negation required to bring herself into line with schemas directing feminine social behavior".[15] Jack's extensive exploratory and longitudinal studies with this group resulted in her development of the STSS, a 31-item, self-rating instrument with four subscales that measure "silencing" behaviors.

• The Externalized Self represents feelings of judging oneself by external standards.
• Care as Self-Sacrifice represents putting the needs of others before the self.
• Silencing the Self (subscale) represents refraining from self-expression and action to avoid conflict and possible loss in the relationship.
• The Divided Self represents the woman who presents with an outer compliant self to fulfill feminine role imperatives while the inner self grows angry and hostile.

19. How is the STSS useful to health care providers?

The knowledge of the different aspects of silencing the self-identified by Jack can help caregivers address interventions that are specific and unique for women.[9,10] In particular, DeMarco et al.[10] found that, of all the silencing behaviors identified by Jack, Care as Self-Sacrifice was demonstrated most frequently. Women would rather take care of the needs of their children at all stages of development before their own needs, especially as they related to their own illness.

In the spirit of family nursing, the considerable silencing behavior related to protection of many women's relationships with their children may be a useful way to reach out to women, not only in adult care settings but also in pediatric settings. Other implications for nursing are simply talking to women about silencing behaviors and how they experience them from a unique cultural, social, or even racial perspective. Women should have the opportunity to start a dialogue about how power structures, including their sexual relationships with men, put them in positions of acquiescing rather than choosing safe sex behaviors or how the use of chemical substances can blur the strength of their voice in asking for what they want and need or just saying "no."

BIBLIOGRAPHY

1. American Academy of Pediatrics: Female genital mutilation. Pediatrics 102:153–156, 1998.
2. Anderson J (ed): A Guide to the Clinical Care of Women with HIV. Washington, DC, Health Resources and Services Administration, 2000.
3. Bellamy C: Helping young women fight sexism and HIV. Boston Globe, December 1, 2000.
4. Brady M: Female genital mutilation: Complications and risk of HIV transmission. AIDS Patient Care STDS 13(12):709–716, 1999.
5. Bruneau J, et al: Sex-specific determinants of HIV infection among injection drug users in Montreal. Cam Med Assoc J/J Assoc Med Can 164(6):767–773, 2001.
6. Centers for Disease Control and Prevention: US HIV and AIDS cases reported through June 2000. HIV/AIDS Surveillance Report, 12 (1), 2000. Available at www.cdc.gov/hiv/stats/hasr1201/table7.htm.
7. Centers for Disease Control and Prevention: Basic statistics—International statistics. Available at http://www.cdc.gov/hiv/stats/internat.htm. Accessed 8/22/01.
8. Cohen M, et al: Domestic violence and childhood sexual abuse in HIV-infected women and women at risk for HIV. Am J Public Health 90:560–565, 2000.
9. DeMarco RF, et al: From silencing the self to action: Experiences of women living with HIV/AIDS. Health Care Women Int 19:539–552, 1998.
10. DeMarco RF, et al: Content validity of a scale to measure silencing and affectivity among women living with HIV/AIDS. J Assoc Nurses AIDS Care 12(4):77–88, 2001.
11. Freidemann ML: The Framework of Systemic Organization: A Conceptual Approach to Families and Nursing. Thousand Oaks, CA, Sage, 1995.
12. Gilligan C: In a Different Voice: Psychological Theory and Women's Development. Cambridge, MA, Harvard University Press, 1982.
13. Gollub EL, et al: Gender differences in risk behaviors among HIV+ persons with an IDU history. The link between partner characteristics and women's higher drug-sex risks. The Manif 2000 Study Group. Sex Trans Dis 25(9): 483–488, 1998.
14. Hader SL, et al: HIV infection in women in the United States: Status at the millennium. JAMA 285:1186–1192, 2001.
15. Jack DC: Silencing the Self: Women and Depression. New York, Harper Collins, 1991.
16. Susser I, Stein Z: Culture, sexuality, and women's agency in the prevention of HIV/AIDS in Southern Africa. Am J Public Health 90:1042–1048, 2000.
17. Williams HA: A comparison of social support and social networks of black parents and white parents with chronically ill children. Soc Sci Med 37:1509–1520, 1993.

19. PREGNANCY AND HIV/AIDS

Sandra A. Averitt, PhD, RN, LCCE, and
Richard L. Sowell, PhD, RN, FAAN

Because of the scientific advances that have been made in developed countries worldwide during the past decade, the relatively low risk of vertical transmission of HIV/AIDS from mother to fetus has dramatically influenced the decision-making process of both health care providers and women infected with HIV. A recent study of reproductive issues for women with HIV found that among 33 women who were either previously unsure or not planning to become pregnant, "the ability to decrease vertical transmission could affect future pregnancy plans."[12] Women who previously believed they had no choice regarding the decision to become pregnant are now making the decision in favor of pregnancy. With this background in mind, it is important for health care providers to be informed and to provide accurate information about the risks of pregnancy and to assist women with reproductive decision-making. Although interaction among a complex set of psychosocial factors plays a part in women's reproductive choices, factors related to health status must also be considered.

1. What factors influence women's decisions to become pregnant once they are diagnosed with HIV infection?

HIV-infected women face many of the same issues related to reproductive decision-making as other women. However, they also face the possibility that they may pass HIV (via perinatal transmission) to their infants. Although HIV seropositive status can be a factor in a woman's decision to become pregnant or terminate a pregnancy, research has shown that HIV status is often not the deciding factor.[3,11,18,22,28,36] For women with the dual diagnosis of HIV and substance use, who exchange sex for money or drugs, the decision may not be whether to have a baby but rather whether to continue an unplanned pregnancy. For other HIV-infected women, many psychosocial factors beyond health status affect their decision-making.

Health care professionals who work with HIV-infected women of reproductive age must fully understand the significance of motherhood to women. For many women, motherhood is steeped in cultural and social meaning. The act of becoming a mother defines the woman as an adult and establishes her place in the community or cultural group.[31,40] Motherhood can be the source of obtaining meaning in life as well as leaving a legacy for the future. In addition, the importance placed on family and the desires of a husband or primary sex partner for children can influence women's desire for a baby.[35] A study of HIV-infected women in the South found that the significant other (husbands and sex partners) and family members were important in women's decisions to have a baby.[36] The support of family in making the decision takes on greater importance for women with HIV infection compared with many other women because it is necessary to consider who will care for the infant/child if the woman becomes ill or dies.

Furthermore, women who hold more traditional beliefs about their gender role and/or do not have other children may be more likely to want a baby. Even when dealing with illness related to HIV, some women see a baby as a positive influence on their lives and believe that the baby will give them someone to love.[36]

Although a number of factors other than HIV infection have been shown to influence women's reproductive decisions, it is important to remember that HIV-infected women are individuals. Without an assessment of a woman's beliefs and life situation it is impossible to determine the exact array of factors that will guide her decision to have a baby or continue a pregnancy.

2. What are the recommendations when a discordant couple (one HIV-infected partner and one uninfected partner) makes the decision to have a baby?

The issue of discordant couples underscores the importance of people knowing their HIV status, even though they may not believe that they are at risk for HIV infection. As HIV infection becomes more widespread in the heterosexual community, the number of discordant couples will increase. Recommendations about approaches to becoming pregnant may depend on the gender and health status of the infected partner. Counseling serodiscordant couples is key to ensuring that they are knowledgeable about the risks and options associated with the decision to become pregnant so that they can make the best decision for their individual situation.

A second factor that needs to be considered, whether the infected partner is male or female, is the level of HIV-RNA, also known as viral load. The goal of treatment is to decrease the level of virus circulating in a person's blood. Low (or undetectable) viral load is believed to be of significant benefit to the couple who desires pregnancy because the lower the viral load in the blood, the less chance of transmission during sexual activity. Although this principle may be generally true, some evidence indicates that the concentration of virus may vary from one body fluid to another. Therefore, an undetectable viral load in the blood does not guarantee that HIV cannot be transmitted through semen or vaginal fluids.[30] However, it is generally accepted that attaining a low viral load is an important step when discordant couples are considering approaches to pregnancy.

3. What are the recommendations when the male partner is HIV-positive and the woman is uninfected?

Male-to-female transmission is more likely than female-to-male transmission. Therefore, when the male partner is HIV-infected, a more rigorous approach is necessary to protect the health of the female partner. Currently, variations on "sperm washing," artificial insemination, and in vitro fertilization are being used to assist HIV-negative women in getting pregnant when their partners are HIV-positive. "Sperm washing" is a procedure in which sperm are collected from the male and then cleansed to remove the HIV virus. This procedure is thought to be effective because the virus is present in the semen but does not appear to infect the sperm directly.[14] After the cleansing procedure, the sperm are inseminated into the woman at the time of ovulation, with the hope of impregnation. This procedure minimizes the risk of HIV transmission to the female partner. In a more experimental procedure under investigation, sperm are isolated from a semen specimen by centrifuge, cleansed of virus, cryopreserved, and then used to fertilize the ovum through in vitro technology. Successful fertilization results in an embryo that can then be implanted into the female. Needless to say, these procedures are complicated and expensive, requiring both psychological and financial commitment by the couple. Such a commitment may not be realistic for the couple, and access to such technologies may be limited. The question of whether the risks of having unprotected sex are high enough to warrant such efforts should be dealt with honestly. Despite the potential effectiveness of highly active antiretroviral therapy (HAART), artificial insemination may further minimize risk.[14]

4. What are the recommendations when the woman is HIV-positive and her partner is uninfected?

A growing body of evidence indicates that transmission from a positive female to a negative male is less likely. Nonetheless, couples must understand that there is always some degree of risk of HIV transmission from the female to the male partner. The safest approach for impregnation is obviously artificial insemination of sperm from the male partner. For those who are unwilling or unable to use this approach and who desire a more natural approach to impregnation, the goal is to limit exposure of the male to the woman's vaginal secretions, which may contain high levels of virus. The first recommendation is for the woman to undergo therapy to reduce the viral load to the lowest level possible. Undetectable levels of virus (HIV-RNA) decrease the risk of transmission to approximately 1%.[14] Decreased viral load is important not only in considering pregnancy but also in the prevention of perinatal transmission. Once the viral load is decreased, the aim is to time any episodes of unprotected sex to coincide with the woman's ovulatory cycle to limit even further the man's exposure.

5. What are the chances that an HIV-infected woman will pass the virus to her infant via perinatal transmission?

A number of situation-specific factors can influence the chances that a woman will transmit HIV to the fetus during pregnancy. It is generally estimated that without treatment 14–40% of the infants born to HIV-infected mothers will be infected.[4,45] These rates vary depending on the region of the world in which the mother lives and the availability of supportive health care. The highest rates of perinatal transmission (without treatment) are in resource-limited countries such as those in southern Africa. The lowest transmission rates have been reported in Western Europe. It is commonly held to be true that the greater the viral load (HIV-RNA), the lower the CD4 counts, and the more advanced the maternal disease process, the greater the incidence of perinatal transmission.[34]

However, research in the early 1990s showed that treatment of the mother during pregnancy with antiretroviral therapy could significantly lower the potential of HIV transmission to the infant. The Pediatric AIDS Clinical Trial Group (PACTG) Protocol 076 demonstrated that treatment of the mother with zidovudine (AZT) during pregnancy, followed by the short-term treatment of the infant after birth, could reduce the perinatal transmission by approximately 66%.[9,10,30]

Further advances in the use of combination therapies have reduced transmission rates to as low as 1%.[30] Current patient management strategies, including good perinatal care, successful management of viral load, and proactive delivery methods, have the potential for further decreasing the rate of transmission.

6. What factors should be considered by health care providers when advising HIV-infected women about pregnancy decisions?

Factors to be considered in advising HIV-infected women about pregnancy include the following:

- Stage of disease progression (CD4 and viral load)
- Use of antiretroviral therapy
- Maternal factors such as drug/ and alcohol abuse
- Other health issues (e.g., hypertension, diabetes, opportunistic infection)
- Maternal age
- Future plans for the care of the child(ren) if the mother's condition deteriorates

Interestingly, studies have shown that significant survival benefit is linked to clinician expertise. Therefore, women with HIV must be under the care of a clinician who is well versed in the management of HIV. When the clinician is faced with advising the woman about pregnancy options, it may become necessary to involve a practitioner who has expertise in obstetrics as part of the management team. As previously discussed, the lower the viral load and the higher the percentage of CD4s, the less likely that vertical transmission will occur. It is important, however, to be sure that the woman understands that there have been documented cases of vertical transmission despite undetectable viral loads.

The use of antiretroviral therapy must be decided on a case-by-case basis, depending on the health and desires of the woman. If the woman has an undetectable viral load, the recommendation of the clinician may be to delay therapy, at least until after the first trimester when teratogenic effects on the fetus are less likely to occur. Nausea and vomiting, common in the first trimester, may eliminate the feasibility of using some antiretrovirals in certain women. If the woman is already on an antiretroviral regimen, the clinician must evaluate the risks and benefits of her regimen in light of the potential pregnancy.[30]

Other concerns related to the mother's health, such as substance abuse or comorbidities, need to be factored into management and counseling. Issues surrounding substance abuse, such as lack of adherence to prescribed medical regimens, engaging in risky behaviors, and decreased self-care, have implications for the health of the fetus as well as the mother. When substance abuse is documented or suspected, the practitioner must address this issue in both counseling about pregnancy and referral for appropriate treatment before conception, if possible. When other health problems exist, the risks associated with pregnancy need to be addressed. When a woman is already pregnant, these health problems need to be considered in establishing a plan of care.[5]

In all women, risks of pregnancy increase with advanced maternal age. Older women with HIV should be advised to consider these risks. The clinician must consider that the motivation for pregnancy may be stronger for a woman who has no children compared with a woman who already has a child. The practitioner must be sensitive to the importance of motherhood to many women. The clinician also needs to be aware that his or her role is that of counselor and advisor. Ultimately women make the decision to become pregnant whether they remain in care or not. The best therapeutic modality is to respect the woman's decision and to develop a partnership in care planning that promotes the best possible outcome for mother and fetus.

7. How does becoming pregnant affect the disease progression of HIV-infected women?

Numerous studies have examined the affect of pregnancy on the progression of HIV disease. All studies to date indicate that pregnancy has no adverse effects on the course of HIV.[5,14,44] The normal hemodilution that occurs as a result of the increased plasma blood volume of pregnancy may result in some drop in absolute CD4 counts; however, the percentage of CD4 cells remains stable, and HIV-RNA counts tend to remain stable throughout pregnancy.[5]

8. What recommendations should be made to HIV-infected women who are contemplating pregnancy and taking multiple-drug therapy?

Multiple-drug therapy is not considered a contraindication for becoming pregnant. It is necessary to consult a clinician to determine the best combination of drugs with the least risk of teratogenic effects,[41] preferably before conception. Sometimes the woman must add to her treatment regimen a drug or drugs that have been shown to have a higher potential to decrease perinatal transmission in order to optimize pregnancy outcome. The woman must understand that the arbitrary discontinuation of one or more of the drugs can result in drug resistance and rebound of viral load levels. Rebound of viral load has negative implications not only for the woman but also for the fetus. A key to adherence is the thorough education of the woman about the prescribed regimen and an understanding that, if side effects occur, consultation with the clinician is essential before discontinuation of the medication.[30]

9. What factors need to be considered in the decision of HIV-infected women to take antiretroviral medications if they become pregnant?

Two related actions, associated with adequate adherence to medications, need to be considered in talking about women's use of antiretroviral medications to decrease perinatal transmission of HIV. First, women must positively evaluate the use of the medication and make the decision to accept the therapy. Second, women must be willing and able to adhere to the prescribed therapy. A number of psychosocial and personal barriers can influence their willingness to accept and adhere to prescribed therapy. Examples include the poor treatment of women and racial minorities in the health care system, lack of trust in health care professionals, and lack of accurate information.[23,37,43,47] Individual barriers include disclosure issues, responsibility for children and family, inability to focus on self, fear of side effects, and myths about treatment. Research in health psychology, related to accepting and adhering to medications, supports the importance of patient-provider communication and social support in the woman's decision to take medications and follow through with the prescribed regimen.[8,33]

Factors identified as influencing women's decisions to accept antiretroviral therapy include beliefs about the effectiveness of the medication, previous experience with the medication, relationship with health care professionals, and a belief that the primary health care provider was positive about the women taking the medication.[27,38] Many HIV-infected women have taken antiretroviral medications and/or know someone who has taken them. The question is whether they think that the medication works. An important factor in women's evaluation of the medication is accurate information. Women who are pregnant or considering pregnancy must have knowledge about the potential benefits of antiretroviral medications in decreasing perinatal transmission of

HIV. Even when women report that they have knowledge of antiretroviral therapy and under-stand its use, clinicians may need to evaluate this understanding and provide clarification if necessary.[43] The development of a partnership between patients and health care providers cannot be overemphasized. Open communication is necessary for the clinician to fully assess the patient and to prescribe therapy; in addition, the woman's assessment of how the clinician views antiretroviral therapy during pregnancy has been shown to be a significant factor in her decision to accept it.[39]

Multiple-drug therapy for HIV has become the standard of care in the United States. Issues that can influence women's willingness and/or ability to adhere to therapy include the difficulty of the treatment regimen (number of pills and dietary restrictions), side effects, understanding of the importance to remain on therapy, cultural beliefs, social support, physical health, and mental status.[46] Side effects related to antiretroviral therapy and a lack of adequate education about these side effects are significant factors in lack of adherence. This may be a particular issue for women who become pregnant. Side effects such as fatigue, nausea, and vomiting have been reported in some patients who take AZT, which is commonly used to decrease perinatal transmission of HIV. For pregnant women, especially in the first trimester, these symptoms can be a normal part of pregnancy. The use of drug therapy can exacerbate these symptoms, making adherence difficult. Clinicians must educate women about possible side effects of drug therapy and en-courage them to report problems with medications so that they can be managed rather than dis-continue treatment.

10. How can an HIV-infected mother have a baby who is not HIV-infected?

Blood is one of the most infectious of all body fluids. Because the fetus receives nutrients, oxygen, antibodies, and other substances, such as alcohol and/or drugs, through the placental circulation, it might be expected that the fetus would become infected through the maternal blood supply. Although the exact mechanism that protects the fetus is not well understood, it is believed that the placenta forms a barrier between the mother and fetus, usually preventing the passage of the virus to the fetus. Many researchers believe that over 60% of perinatal transmis-sions occur at the time of delivery, further supporting the belief in the protective nature of the placenta.[45]

11. What are the recommendations for treatment of opportunistic infections in pregnant HIV-infected women? Is the treatment a threat to the fetus?

Recommendations for the management of opportunistic infections in pregnancy have been developed by a number of federal agencies through expert panels.[5] All pregnant women with HIV need to be carefully screened and monitored for opportunistic infections. If a woman has had pre-vious opportunistic infections, the recommendation is primary prophylaxis throughout life to avoid infection. Currently, prophylaxis of *Pneumocystis carinii* pneumonia is the same as for the nonpregnant client. The key to the management of all other opportunistic infections is to weigh the risks versus the benefits of the drugs used to treat nonpregnant patients and to substitute agents that, in consultation with experts, are least likely to have an adverse effect on the fetus while effectively treating the mother.

12. Are immunizations appropriate for HIV-infected women during pregnancy?

The effect of immunizations should also be considered when the risk of exposure for the mother and/or fetus is high. HIV-infected people must avoid any vaccines that contain live bacte-ria or live virus. The most commonly recommended vaccines include pneumococcal vaccine, he-patitis B, influenza, enhanced-potency inactivated polio vaccine (not oral), hepatitis A vaccine, and immune globulins when a mother is exposed to measles or varicella.[5] Because of the rapid advancement of research in HIV/AIDS and its treatment, clinicians must be aware of the latest developments in treatment recommendations and guidelines. A number of websites continually update information related to the treatment guidelines for HIV/AIDS, including www.hivatis.org, www.amfar.org/td and www.hab.hrsa.gov.

13. What are the current recommendations for mode of delivery for HIV-infected women?

For women who receive adequate prenatal care and are on HAART or who have low or undetectable viral loads, vaginal delivery may be the best choice. However, a growing body of evidence reports that cesarean section, under some conditions, may be advantageous in preventing perinatal transmission. Conditions in which cesarean section should be considered include rupture of membranes longer than 4 hours, prolonged labor, and/ or high maternal viral load. These conditions have been shown to increase the likelihood of transmission during the birth process. Some clinicians intervene in such circumstances to perform a cesarean section. The Public Health Service Task Force recommends that HIV-1 RNA levels be evaluated at 34–36 weeks' gestation to allow discussion of the optimal mode of delivery based on clinical status and HIV RNA-1 results. In a 2000 position statement, the American College of Obstetrics and Gynecology recommended scheduled cesarean sections for HIV-1 RNA results > 1,000 copies/ml.[30] Women should be provided information about the risks and benefits of both cesarean section and vaginal delivery, recognizing that cesarean section is an operative procedure with an inherent set of risks to both mother and child. Given this information, the decision is ultimately that of the woman in concert with her clinician, and her decision should be respected.[5,14] More research into the benefits of cesarean section needs to be done before it is promoted as the accepted mode of delivery for all women with HIV infection. Regardless of the mode of delivery, there is no guarantee that HIV transmission can be prevented in all cases.

14. What special treatments are recommended for mother and infant in the early postpartum period?

In the early postpartum period, women are at greater risk for hemorrhage secondary to the birth process. In some institutions, methergine (a drug that stimulates uterine contraction) may be administered to control postpartum bleeding. Because a drug interaction may occur between protease inhibitors and ergot derivatives and precipitate coronary vasospasm, other agents should be used to prevent potential complications.[14] In addition, the Food and Drug Administration (FDA) has identified a potentially life-threatening interaction between delavirdine (Rescriptor), a synthetic nonnucleoside reverse transcriptase inhibitor, and ergot derivatives, including methergine, that can result in "acute ergot toxicity with peripheral vasospasm and ischemia of the extremities and other tissues"[13] (pp. 17–18). The need to investigate potential drug interactions thoroughly before administering any drug in conjunction with antiretroviral therapy cannot be stressed enough. Although some drugs may cause minimal side effects, drug interactions can also render certain HIV-specific drugs more or less potent. The FDA provides an excellent website to research drug interactions at http://www.fda.gov.

Assessment of wound healing, proper involution, and postpartum bleeding are important, as with all women after delivery. Women need to be instructed about how to handle and/or dispose of articles exposed to lochia (blood and tissue discharged after birth), such as peripads and clothing. Strategies for lactation suppression, such as compression, nonsteroidal anti-inflammatory drugs (NSAIDs), and ice packs, should be discussed before discharge. Appropriate referral for ongoing management of HIV disease and follow-up with gynecologic care are essential.[5,14] If the woman has substance abuse problems, follow-up treatment through a substance abuse program is essential for the well-being of both mother and infant. It is important to discuss the use of contraception and condoms if the woman plans to resume sexual activity.[5,14]

Women who have received antiretroviral therapy during pregnancy need to be reevaluated after delivery with appropriate testing to determine ongoing need for treatment. If continued therapy is recommended, adherence to the medication regimen must be stressed. Health personnel need to be aware that the stresses of the early postpartum period may make adherence difficult; therefore, referral for ongoing support services may be required to ensure the mother's ability to adhere. Because postpartum depression may occur in women with HIV/AIDS, health care providers need to remain vigilant for signs that indicate a need for counseling and treatment.[30]

15. Should HIV-infected women breast-feed their infants?

In the developing countries where formula and safe water are not readily available to women, breast-feeding may be the only option. Some evidence shows that there is a higher risk of HIV transmission through breast-feeding when women both breast- and bottle-fed infants. Therefore, when formula or safe water is not consistently available, it may be better for women to breast-feed all of the time rather than at intervals. Research in developing countries indicates that at least 14–15% of transmission of HIV from mother to child occurs through breast-feeding. For this reason, it is widely accepted in the United States and other developed countries that breast-feeding is contraindicated.[5,14,45] In addition, recent concerns about the long-term exposure of infants to anti-retroviral drugs through breast milk further supports the avoidance of breast-feeding.[30]

16. Are there any specific risks for infants of HIV-infected women beyond the risk of transmission?

Limited evidence suggests that infants of HIV-infected women may be born prematurely.[29,30] Antiretroviral therapy has been linked to this phenomenon. However, to date, few data are available related to degree of prematurity or the relative numbers in relation to full-term deliveries. Therefore, HIV-infected women should be carefully monitored for pregnancy complications. To date, no evidence indicates that exposure to antiretroviral drugs during pregnancy increases the risk for congenital anomalies.[30]

The infant should be bathed immediately after delivery, condition permitting, to reduce the danger of mucocutaneous exposure. The routine administration of vitamin K should be delayed until the bathing has been accomplished. Infants of HIV-positive women must undergo close pediatric follow-up, both to identify health status and to track health and developmental progress if they were exposed to antiretroviral therapy during pregnancy.[5]

17. Does a positive HIV antibody test at birth mean that the infant will develop HIV/AIDS?

No. All infants born to HIV-infected women have a positive HIV antibody test because they received the mother's antibodies during pregnancy. The presence of antibodies does not mean that the baby is HIV-infected. It is estimated that maternal antibodies clear from the infant by 1 year to 18 months after birth. An HIV-infected infant will develop his or her own antibodies to the virus. Once the mother's antibodies clear from the infant's system, the infant who is not HIV-infected will test HIV antibody-seronegative.

18. What is the most accurate test to determine whether an infant is HIV-infected after birth?

The least accurate method for diagnosing HIV infection in infants is antibody testing (see question 17). As noted above, infants have maternal antibodies at birth. To accurately reflect their HIV status, infants must clear the mother's antibodies and develop immune function that allows production of antibodies to actual infection. A second approach to determining HIV infection in infants is testing for the presence of actual virus or measuring viral load. Infants can be definitively diagnosed as HIV-infected between 1 and 6 months of age using viral diagnostic testing.[17] Several viral testing methods are available, including detection of HIV by culture and DNA or RNA polymerase chain reaction (PCR). HIV-DNA PCR testing is considered the method of choice in infants.[17] However, tests that detect HIV- RNA in plasma may be more sensitive than DNA PCR for early diagnosis of HIV in infants. Current federal guidelines suggest that diagnostic testing be performed within the first 48 hours of life, between 1 and 2 months, and between 3 and 6 months of age. The goal of such testing is the early identification of HIV infection so that aggressive antiretroviral therapy can be implemented when appropriate. It is important to note that HIV viral testing is a more expensive and more complex procedure than antibody testing. Therefore, viral testing may not be available or financially feasible for determining HIV infection in infants born to many women infected with HIV. Clinicians need to consider the benefits of viral testing vs. issues of expense and availability in specific clinical settings.

19. What are the current recommendations for treatment of infants who test positive for HIV?

All infants of HIV-positive mothers, regardless of their status, should receive oral zidovudine (AZT) in the delivery room because even infants who test negative initially can seroconvert if infected intrapartum. The recommended dosage for term infants is 2 mg/kg every 6 hours for the first 6 weeks of life. The current regimen under investigation for preterm infants is 1.5 mg/kg by mouth or intravenously every 12 hours for the first 2 weeks of life, then 2 mg/kg every 8 hours for an additional 2–6 weeks. All infants must have a complete blood count and differential done at birth, because AZT can cause anemia. Anemic infants require close monitoring throughout this 6-week period. Hemoglobin testing should be done on infants at 6–12 weeks to rule out AZT-related hematologic toxicity.[30] In addition, all HIV-exposed infants should receive routine prophylaxis for *Pneumocystis carinii* beginning at 4–6 weeks and continuing through the first year of life or until the infant is proved negative for HIV infection. Once infection is confirmed, more intensive combination therapy should be initiated if the infant demonstrates clinical symptoms or evidence of immunosuppression, regardless of the infant's age or viral load. Clinicians must recognize that the first 12 months of life are a critical period during which HIV-infected infants are at high risk for disease progression.[5]

20. Discuss the prognosis for HIV-infected infants.

The question of prognosis is a difficult one. If the infant survives the first year of life, prognosis appears to be better, especially since the availability of pharmacologic agents that appear to be safe for children has increased over the past decade. According to the most current statistics from the American Academy of Pediatrics (1999), 36–61% of children who were infected during the perinatal period are expected to survive to the age of 13 years. The median survival age is 8.6 to 13 years. Survival is thought to depend on the level of infection (i.e., viral load) at birth. Infants whose HIV viral test is positive at or before 48 hours after birth are considered to have early infection and are believed to have more rapid disease progression.[7,26]

21. If the infant is HIV-positive, what is the health care provider's role in assisting women with issues related to disclosure both to family and later to the child?

A high level of stigma continues to be associated with HIV infection because of its historical identification with marginalized people, including gay men, intravenous drug users, ethnic minorities, and sex workers. These groups experienced high levels of stigma even before the advent of HIV/AIDS. Women often experience even greater stigma than their male counterparts, as a result of societal role expectations for women and a double standard of behavior for men and women.[15,32] Furthermore, women, too, often have been viewed as vectors of HIV transmission to sex partners and children rather than as people suffering from a life-threatening disease.[20]

Although it is necessary for women to disclose their HIV infection to access care, this decision has to be balanced with the potentially negative consequences of disclosure. Numerous cases report that women have experienced negative treatment, violence, and abandonment as a result of disclosing their HIV status.[20,47] As a result, many women fail to disclose HIV infection.[19]

Kimberly, Servovich, and Greene[20] have proposed that the decision to disclose is selective and consists of several steps: adjusting to the diagnosis, assessing disclosure skills, deciding whom to tell, evaluating the recipient's contextual situation, anticipating the recipient's reaction, and having a reason to disclose. There may be a need and opportunity for clinicians to assist women in the disclosure process at each of these steps.

Disclosure of infants' HIV infection can be an even greater challenge for women than simply disclosing their own infection. Disclosure carries the risk of stigmatizing the infant, who may be rejected and/or mistreated by family, friends, or other people in the community. Such concerns are often legitimate and should not be discounted by health care professionals. Health care professionals may be most helpful in assisting women to weigh the advantages and disadvantages of disclosing the infant's HIV infection to specific groups. They also can assist women in gaining the skills necessary to disclose. In addition, clinicians can identify available resources that provide women with options when disclosure of HIV infection results in negative reactions by family, partners, and community members. Attention to providing for the safety of the women and their infants is paramount. Actual disclosure decisions vary, depending on the women's situation. Disclosure may not be the best decision in every situation.

When and how to disclose to a child that he or she is HIV-infected is an individual decision made by the mother based on a variety of factors, including the child's age, cognitive development, psychosocial maturity, family dynamics, and clinical picture. The American Academy of Pediatrics[1] suggests that the nature of the disclosure be geared to the child's cognitive development. A younger child should be given simple explanations of the nature of the illness. As the child matures, he or she should be fully informed of the nature and consequences of the illness and encouraged to participate fully in his or her own care.

Several research studies have indicated that 25–90% of children of school age have not been told that they are HIV-infected.[16,25] When parents and/or health care professionals choose not to disclose HIV status to a child who is cognitively mature enough to participate in self-care, a number of ethical issues are raised. Lack of disclosure denies the child a chance to participate in decision-making about his or her care (autonomy) and limits the ability to prepare psychologically for the consequences of having a life-threatening disease. In addition, if the child reaches puberty without the knowledge of the HIV infection, he or she may unwittingly infect another child through high-risk behaviors.[6]

22. What is the role of the health care professional in assisting HIV-infected mothers in planning for ongoing care of their children if they become ill or die?

In 1999, the American Academy of Pediatrics[2] issued a statement that by the end of the year 2000, 80,000 children and adolescents in the U.S. will be orphaned as a direct result of the AIDS epidemic. What happens to the children in the long term, even if they are not infected? As the disease progresses, women are less able to cope with the responsibilities of raising children and managing their own disease. The mothers must consider what arrangements can be made for children in the event that they are hospitalized or die. It is the responsibility of the health care professional to initiate discussion of such issues early in the disease process. State regulations about guardianship vary. If women do not have HIV-negative partners or family members who will assume responsibility for their children, other potential caretakers need to be identified who will provide love and nurturing as well as a stable, consistent environment for the children. This topic needs to be approached with sensitivity since guilt, denial, and fear can hamper future planning efforts. It is important to stress to the women the need to provide a legal framework to protect their children's right to medical care, mental health support for coping with the loss of their parent, and educational needs. Efforts can be further compounded by the fear that disclosure may lead to social ostracism for both parents and children or even the potential loss of custody of the children, especially when drug dependence is involved. Once legal guardians are appointed by the court as agents for the children, the parents lose their parental rights. A few states have instituted "stand-by" guardianship that allows guardians to take over the care of the children during hospitalization and returns custody to the parents if they recover sufficiently to provide care. Foster care does not appear to be a viable option to provide intermittent care.[2]

King[21] describes a model program called Family Options, a custody-planning program administered through the Department of Child and Family Services in the state of Illinois that provides for standby adoption or standby or short-term guardianship. Standby adoption allows the entire adoption process to proceed without terminating parental rights until such time as the parents are unable to function in the parenting role, either through terminal illness or death. This program provides the avenue for a smooth transition for the children while allowing the biologic parent to continue parenting until no longer able. Standby guardianship allows the parents to designate, through court proceedings, the legal guardians in the event that they are unable to function in the parenting role, again without relinquishing parental rights. Short-term guardianship is a temporary transfer of guardianship for a 60-day period when mothers require hospitalization or drug treatment. The major issue with this option is that, in the event of the mothers' death, the children could be without a legal guardian.

Because all of these options take time to implement (between 8 months and 2 years), health care providers must begin the process as early as possible after diagnosis. King[21] identifies four stages of the Family Options Program: outreach and education, developing a permanency plan, securing a court-ordered plan, and aftercare to resolve any family conflicts (p. 1). Health care providers for women infected with HIV must be proactive, both in preparing women for this critical decision-making process and in promoting legislation in their states that allows optimal arrangements for the ongoing care of children affected by HIV/AIDS.

BIBLIOGRAPHY

1. American Academy of Pediatrics: Disclosure of illness status to children and adolescents with HIV infection (RE9827). Pediatrics 103(1):164–166, 1999.
2. American Academy of Pediatrics: Planning for children whose parents are dying of HIV/AIDS (RE9816). Pediatrics 103(2):509–511, 1999.
3. Ahluwalia IB, DeVellis RF, Thomas JC: Reproductive decisions of women at risk for acquiring HIV infection. AIDS Educ Prevent 10(1):90–97, 1988.
4. Anastos K, Denenbery R, Solomon L: Clinical management of HIV-infected women. In Wormser GP (ed): Aids and Other Manifestations of HIV Infection, 3rd ed., Philadelphia, Lippincott, 1998, pp 339–348.
5. Anderson J: HIV and reproduction. In A Guide to the Clinical Care of Women with HIV. Washington, DC, U.S. Department of Health and Human Services, Health Resources and Services Administration, HIV/AIDS Bureau, 2001, pp 213-274. Available at http://www.hab.hrsa.gov/.
6. Boatner L: To tell or not to tell: The ethics of disclosure in pediatric AIDS by vertical transmission. J Assoc Nurses AIDS Care 13(2):64–66, 2002.
7. Bryson YJ, Luzuriaga K, Sullivan JL, Wara DW: Proposed definitions for in utero versus intrapartum transmission of HIV-1. N Engl J Med 327:1246–1247, 1993.
8. Burke L, Dunbar-Jacobs J: Adherence to medication, diet, and activity recommendations: From assessment to maintenance. J Clin Nurs 9(2):62–79, 1995.
9. Centers for Disease Control and Prevention: Birth outcomes following zidovudine therapy in pregnant women. MMWR 42:409, 415–416, 1994.
10. Connor EM, Sperling RS, Belber R, et al: Reduction of maternal-infant transmission of human immunodeficiency virus type-1 with zidovudine treatment. N Engl J Med 331:462–477, 1993.
11. Cremieux N, Mandelbrot L, Firtion G, et al: HIV-seropositive pregnant women's choice to deliver or to terminate pregnancy. Proceedings of the International Conference on AIDS 9(1):462–477, 1993.
12. Duggan J, Walerius H, Purohit A, et al: Reproductive issues in HIV-seropositive women: A survey regarding counseling, contraception, safer sex, and pregnancy choices. J Assoc Nurses AIDS Care 10(5):84–92, 1999.
13. Food and Drug Administration: Rescriptor-NDA 20-705/S-008. Medwatch 4-37, 2001. Available at http://www.fda.gov.
14. Garcia P: Reproductive choice for HIV-affected women: What does it really mean? In Women and HIV: The Continuing Challenge. Chicago, Northwestern University Medical School, Medical Chicago Education Collaborative, 2000, pp 1–6. Available at http://www.medscape.com/Medscape/HIV/TreatmentUpdate/2000.
15. Grove KA, Kelly DP, Liu J: But nice girls don't get it: Women, symbolic capital, and the social construct of AIDS. J Clin Epidemiol 26:317–337, 1997.
16. Grubman S, Gross E, Lerner-Weiss N, et al: Older children and adolescents living with perinatally acquired human immunodeficiency virus infection. Pediatrics 95:657–663, 1995.
17. Guidelines for the Use of Antiretroviral Agents in Pediatric HIV Infection. Developed by NPHRC, HRSA, and NIH, December 14, 2001, pp 1–68. Available at www.hivatis.org.
18. Johnstone FD, Brettle RP, MacCallum LR, et al: Women's knowledge of their HIV antibody state: Its effects on their decision whether to continue the pregnancy. Br Med J 300(6):23–36, 1990.
19. Kalichman SC, Nachimson D: Self-efficacy and disclosure of HIV-positive serostatus to sex partners. Health Psychol 18:281–287, 1999.
20. Kimberly JA, Serovich JM, Greene K: Disclosure of HIV-positive status: Five women's stories. Fam Relat 44:316–322, 1995.
21. King E: Custody and Permanency Planning. Women and HIV: The Continuing Challenge, 1-2, 2000. Available at http://www.medscape.com/medscape/HIV/Treatment Update/2000.
22. Kline A, Strickler J, Kempf J: Factors associated with pregnancy and pregnancy resolution in HIV seropositive women. Social Sci Med 40:1539–1547, 1995.
23. Lancioni C, Harwell T, Rutstein RM: Prenatal care and HIV infection. AIDS Patient Care STDs 13:97–102, 1999.
24. Lindegren ML, Byers RH, Thomas P, et al: Trends in perinatal transmission of HIV/AIDS in the United States. JAMA 282:531–538, 1999.
25. Lipson M: Disclosure of diagnosis to children with human immunodeficiency virus or acquired immunodeficiency syndrome. J Devel Behav Pediatr 15:s61–s65, 1994.
26. Mayaux M. J, Burgard M, Teglas JP, et al: Neonatal characteristics in rapidly progressive perinatally acquired HIV-1 disease. JAMA 275:606–610, 1996.

27. Misener RT, Sowell RL: HIV-infected women's decisions to take antiretrovirals. West J Nurs Res 20(4):431–447, 1998.
28. Murphy DA, Mann T, O'Keefe Z, Rotheram-Borus MJ: Number of pregnancies, outcome expectancies, and social norms among HIV-infected young women. Health Psychol 17(5):470–475, 1998.
29. Newell M: Combination anti-HIV therapy during pregnancy ups risk of premature delivery. AIDS 2000 14:2913–2920, 2001.
30. Public Health Service Task Force Recommendations for Use of Antiretroviral Drugs in Pregnant HIV-1-Infected Women for Maternal Health and Interventions to Reduce Perinatal HIV-1 Transmission in the United States, February 4, 2002, pp 1–46. Available at http://www.hivais.org.
31. Pivnic A: Loss and regeneration: Influences on the reproductive decisions of HIV positive, drug-using women. Med Anthropol 16:39–62, 1994.
32. Pizzi M: Women, HIV infection, and AIDS tapestries of life, death, and empowerment. Am J Occup Ther 46:1021–1027, 1992.
33. Rheiner NW: A theoretical framework for research on client compliance with a rehabilitation program. Rehabil Nurs Res 4(3):90–97, 1995.
34. Smith KY: Can I have children? AIDS Care 2(4), 1998. Available at http://www/hivnewsline.com.
35. Sowell RL, Phillips KD, Misener T: HIV-infected women and motivation to add children to their family. J Fam Nurs 5(3):316–331, 1999.
36. Sowell RL, Misener T: Decisions to have a baby by HIV-infected women. West J Nurs Res 19(1):56–70, 1997.
37. Sowell RL, Seals B, Moneyham L, et al: Barriers and health seeking behaviors of women infected with HIV. Nurs Conn 9(3):5–17, 1996.
38. Sowell RL, Phillips KD, Murdaugh C, et al: Health care providers' influence on HIV-infected women's beliefs and intentions related to AZT therapy. Clin Nurs Res 8(4):336–354, 1999.
39. Sowell RL, Phillips KD, Seals BF, et al: HIV-Infected women's experiences and beliefs related to AZT therapy during pregnancy. AIDS Patient Care STDs 15(4):201–209, 2001.
40. Sunderland A: Influence of human immunodeficiency virus infection on reproductive decisions. Obstet Gynecol Clin North Am 17:585–593, 1990.
41. Tabers' Cyclopedic Medical Dictionary, 19th ed. Philadelphia, F.A. Davis, 2001.
42. Turnstal CG, Kegeles S, Downing M, Darney P: Women at high risk for perinatal HIV transmission: Risk profiles by reproductive lifestage, HIV serostatus and race/ethnicity. Proceedings of the International Conference on AIDS [abstract no. PoC4655]. 1992.
43. USPHS/IDSA Guidelines for the Prevention of Opportunistic Infections in Person Infected with Human Immunodeficiency Virus. 2001, pp 1–64. Available at http://www.hivatis.org/guidelines.
44. Vitiello MA, Smeltzer SC: HIV, pregnancy, and zidovudine: What do women know? J Assoc Nurses AIDS Care 10:41–47, 1991.
45. Weisser M, Rudin C, Battegay M, et al: Does pregnancy influence the course of HIV infection? J AIDS 17:404–410, 1998.
46. Wilfert CM: A call to action. HIV Newsline 6(1),1-4, February, 2000. Available at http://www.hivnewsline.com/issues.
47. Williams A: Antiretroviral therapy: Factors associated with adherence. J Assoc Nurses AIDS Care 8(Supp 1):18–23, 1997.
48. Yep GA: Disclosure of HIV infection interpersonal relationships: A communication boundary management approach. In: Petronnio S (ed): Balancing the Secrets of Private Disclosures. Mahwah, NJ, Laurence Erlbaum Associates, 2000, pp 83–96.

20. THE ELDERLY AND HIV/AIDS

Judy K. Shaw, MS, ACRN, ANP-C

The elderly have not always been considered a population at risk or a focus of HIV prevention messages—in part because of the myth in Western Society that only young, attractive, and healthy people are sexually active. In fact, in 1997 the Centers for Disease Control and Prevention (CDC) released surveillance statistics that identified the 50+ age group as having the greatest percentage increase in AIDS cases.[1] After the release of that information, interventions have been developed to focus on prevention efforts aimed at older adults.

1. How many older people have HIV/AIDS?

In their latest surveillance statistics, the CDC estimated that about 84,000 U.S. cases were people age 50+ at the time of diagnosis with AIDS. The greatest incidence occurred in people ages 50–54. The majority of those infected are Caucasian men (34,540), followed by African American (24,665) and Hispanic (11,414) men. Most cases in women are among African Americans (6,605), followed by Caucasians (3,378) and Hispanics (2,471). Overall, these cases account for about 22% of the total U.S. population with AIDS. Estimates including persons with HIV infection are even greater. For example, the CDC[2] reported a total of about 320,000 persons living with AIDS in the U.S at the end of 2000. However, at the same time an estimated 850,000 people in the U.S. are living with HIV infection.

2. Why is there a difference between estimates of HIV infection and reported cases of AIDS?

First, HIV disease simply means infection with the HIV virus. AIDS is defined as a CD4 cell count ≤ 200 in the presence of the HIV virus and/or the presence of an AIDS-defining illness.

Until recently, most states required only that the number of cases of AIDS be reported because of the stigma related to HIV/AIDS infection. These numbers were mainly used for epidemiologic records and support of funding. Unlike syphilis or other reportable communicable diseases, the names of people newly diagnosed with HIV were not reported to the state departments of health. Even now, not all states require name reporting when a diagnosis is confirmed, and many agencies continue to offer anonymous testing. In fact, for every known case of AIDS, there are possibly another 2–3 cases of HIV infection. Using this formula, as many as 225,000 people in the 50+ age group may be living with HIV/AIDS infection in the U.S.

An understanding of this information is important because the number of AIDS cases has declined overall since the advent of antiretroviral therapy. Reports in the media have given a false feeling of security to many people who think that HIV is also on the decline. What has been on the decline for the past few years, at least in the United States, is the number of cases of HIV that have progressed to meet the AIDS criteria. In other developing countries, such is not the case. This false sense of security has prompted a resurgence of unsafe sexual practices among many groups; in fact, HIV infection has been reported to be on the rise in the gay community.

3. How do older people become infected with HIV?

Older adults have the same risk factors as their younger counterparts. The most common route of HIV infection in people age 50+ in the U.S. is unprotected sexual exposure. The greatest incidence is reported among men who have sex with men (32.5%).[1] Injection drug use and heterosexual activity are the next most likely routes. Many older persons are not able to identify a route of infection. In one recent study,[3] almost one-fifth (19.3%) of participants reported not knowing for sure how they were infected. This situation highlights the need for HIV education in the 50+ age group. Especially important is the use of barriers for all sexual encounters. Older adults, who are less likely to know the possible routes of HIV infection, often consider the use of barriers to be specific for preventing pregnancy. Even if they acknowledge the need for condoms with unknown partners, they are less likely to realize that HIV can be transmitted through vaginal, pre-ejaculation, and seminal fluid, making barriers necessary for safe oral sex as well. Although much less risky, sharing toothbrushes and razors can also put someone at risk for HIV infection.

HIV has become endemic among older adults in areas where large proportions of retirees live, such as the states of Florida and Arizona. Many of the residents of "retirement communities" are single and, intending to enjoy their freedom, may not be in monogamous relationships. In this setting, the likelihood of infection increases, especially if sex for money takes place. Retirees often travel home for the spring and summer and become conduits for infection.

4. Why does HIV/AIDS education have to be specifically targeted at elderly people?

Many of the early HIV prevention messages were developed to appeal to groups considered to be at high risk for infection, including gay men, drug users, and people with multiple sexual partners. Content included the risks involved with unprotected sex with unknown or multiple partners, sharing needles, and people having sex for money and/or drugs. Older people interpreted this information to mean that, since they were not engaging in sex with prostitutes or using heroin, they were safe. In fact, many "tuned out" the messages, feeling that HIV was a disease of people with deviant lifestyles. Condoms are considered a form of birth control rather than a protective barrier for sexually transmitted disease among the elderly, who are beyond the age for conception and, therefore, do not routinely use condoms.

In fact, most people aged 50+ do not engage in high-risk behaviors and so are correct in not seeing themselves at risk.[4] Persons identified as having risky behaviors are unlikely to change.[5]

Since the release of the CDC statistics, new interventions have been developed focusing on the unique needs of the elderly. Promotion materials featuring older adults are used to capture the attention of the elderly and to provide information about why they need to practice safe behaviors. Older adults with HIV have also captured the attention of the media. Shortly after the release of the 1997 CDC statistics,[1] articles highlighting the increased incidence of HIV among the elderly appeared in national newspapers and magazines and were featured on national broadcasts on television. Programs were developed, and older adults, especially from minority populations, were trained as peer counselors and spokespersons to spread the message to their fellow senior citizens.

5. Are the elderly sexually active?

The majority of men (71%) and women (51%) age 60+ who participated in a survey conducted in 1988 by the National Council on Aging indicated that they were still sexually active. Becoming older does not mean that people do not need to feel loved and wanted by the opposite (or same) sex. In fact, people of retirement age may feel less conflict from work-related stress and be more able to focus on personal needs. Advances in technology have changed the way that people age. In the previous century, people living past 50 were considered old. Now people in the eighth or ninth decade of life are living active and productive lives. Sexual activity among the elderly may be in part a response to overall improvements in quality of life and health.

6. What are some of the differences between younger and older persons with HIV/AIDS?

Older people with HIV/AIDS are much more likely to be diagnosed later in the course of the disease. Because older adults are not considered to be a group at high risk, an HIV test is often not ordered until other age-related conditions have been ruled out as a diagnosis. For example, when an older person is admitted to the hospital for pneumonia, providers are more likely to consider common pathogens rather than HIV. If the source of infection cannot be identified from routine test results (blood and sputum cultures), the provider will look for possible alternatives.

A thorough sexual history is the key factor leading to a diagnosis of HIV/AIDS. Providers may not include this component in the initial exam if the patient is elderly and presents with symptoms that indicate a classic case of community-acquired pneumonia. Other conditions that may be considered age-specific can also be indicators of HIV/AIDS infection:

- Pancytopenia
- Recurrent fungal infections
- Wasting
- Anemia

- Varicella zoster virus
- Non-Hodgkin's lymphoma
- Dementia

In many ways, HIV can be considered an imposter disease because it mimics conditions that are associated with the natural course of aging.

Older people diagnosed with HIV/AIDS may have a poorer prognosis than younger people—due in part to the presence of comorbid conditions. In addition, a natural decrease in immune function is associated with aging, probably due to an inability to replace T cells. Older patients also may be limited in their choice of antiretroviral therapy, if they are taking other medications that have an interaction, such as anticoagulants, hyperlipidemic agents, H_2 blockers, sildenafil, or zolpidem (Ambien).

Older people have less knowledge about HIV/AIDS than younger people. Many believe that they can be infected with HIV/AIDS by being coughed on or using a public toilet.[6] This misunderstanding is a concern for prevention but also contributes to the fear and isolation among the elderly living with HIV/AIDS. They do not want to take a chance of spreading the virus to others whom they know and love and, since they may not have up-to-date knowledge, they withdraw at a time when social support is most needed.

Many younger people already have friends or family members who are HIV-infected and may be familiar with the community resources that are available. Older people are less likely to know others who are infected (in part due to the low overall incidence rate) and are less familiar with the HIV community-based organizations. Even after being informed about the availability of these resources, they are less likely to become involved because of a fear of exposure.

7. Should a sexual history be included in every exam?

A thorough sexual history can provide key information in trying to determine a diagnosis. Because of financial pressures in the health care system, providers' schedules are often overbooked, and they must focus on the presenting complaint and symptoms. It may be a stretch to consider a full history necessary in someone presenting with a cough. For this reason, the nurse plays an important role in triaging the patient. The nurse has the opportunity to ask about recent changes in lifestyle, travel, or unusual symptoms and to report them to the provider.

Another misconception is that married people are not at risk for infection. Although this assumption is probably true if the relationship remains monogamous, spouses have been infected when one partner is engaged in an extramarital relationship with someone at risk. This situation makes a diagnosis difficult, since there are no obvious risk factors.

Older adults may be hesitant to mention behaviors that they feel are deviant to providers, especially if they live in a small or rural town and are concerned about patient confidentiality. Some patients who are living with HIV drive miles to a more urban area to see providers and/or purchase medications rather than risk exposure in their community.

8. Why are older people likely to progress to AIDS more rapidly than younger people with HIV?

Older people have a natural decrease in immune function that some experts believe is related to their inability to replace T cells, an integral part of the immune system.[6] In addition, cytokine production patterns in older adults may result in less effective responses to HIV. Initially, researchers indicated that older adults progress to AIDS more rapidly than younger people diagnosed with HIV, but since the advent of combination antiretroviral therapy, this assumption has been under debate.[6,7] In several studies, antiretroviral therapy was the only independent predictor of survival among the elderly after a diagnosis with AIDS.[6,8]

The second important factor that influences progression to AIDS is stage of disease at diagnosis. Because older adults have traditionally not been seen as a population at high risk, they are more likely to be tested for HIV during hospitalization or after diagnosis of an opportunistic infection. Many have already progressed to AIDS when diagnosed. In either case, the patient may already be severely immunosuppressed. Delayed or no antiretroviral treatment has been identified as a predictor of negative outcomes and/or death.[8] Comorbid conditions may also contribute to a generalized decline in health among the elderly and a decrease in immune function.

9. What is the effect on disease progression of other medical conditions in the elderly?

Comorbid conditions can affect disease progression in HIV. Many older adults have some form of heart disease, diabetes, renal insufficiency, liver disease, or pulmonary disease. Renal and liver diseases are especially important to consider because medications are metabolized through these organs. Antiretroviral therapy may need to be adjusted, depending on how well the kidney and liver are functioning.

Possible drug interactions are also a concern for people who are being treated for comorbid conditions. Regular review of medications is important to ensure that they are taken at the correct dose and time and that patients follow all directions specific for each medication. Patients should be asked about side effects at all visits. Identifying possible side effects in advance helps the patient understand which symptoms may be caused by antiretovirals in contrast to other medications or the effect of aging. Time should be allowed to discuss any possible dietary interactions as well as the use of over-the-counter (OTC) medications and/or complementary therapies.

Many older adults do not realize that OTC medications can have potentially serious side effects. The nurse should remind them to ask at the pharmacy or check with their provider before using any new medication, herbal supplement, or OTC remedy. Older patients often seen multiple specialists for comorbid conditions, and providers may not be aware of all of the medications that are taken. Medication cards that can be presented at visits to all providers ensure that patients have a comprehensive, up-to-date list of all medications and allows thorough examination for possible drug interactions.

10. Is adherence an important part of HIV/AIDS treatment in the elderly?

Adherence is the key factor for successful medical treatment. The elderly should be included in adherence programs and monitored regularly. Medication does not work if it is not taken or if it is taken incorrectly.

All patients should have a part in planning their therapy. Pill burden, dosing schedules, and dietary restrictions must be considered before antiretroviral therapy is started. If the patients show indications of forgetfulness, a simple regimen is best, even if scientifically it may not be the first choice. Devices such as pill boxes and large lettering can be helpful in allowing older patients to maintain their independence with medication self-administration.

Occasionally, unwanted side effects make medication adherence difficult. Diarrhea, nausea, vomiting, and/or rashes must be addressed if the patient is expected to continue therapy. Rashes are always a concern and warrant a provider visit. With some medications therapy must be stopped if a rash develops to prevent dangerous and life-threatening sequelae. Nausea, vomiting, and diarrhea can lead to dehydration and weight loss if untreated. In many cases, these symptoms resolve spontaneously in several days to weeks after a new medication is started. In other cases, when severe symptoms persist, the therapy may have to be changed.

As with other patients with a diagnosis of HIV, fear of stigma and exposure may influence adherence. Patients who have not disclosed their HIV status may be hesitant to take medications in public places (e.g., church, social functions) or to have medications in obvious spots (e.g., medicine cabinets) in their home, where they may be identified or prompt questions from onlookers.

11. What are the age-related differences in the way that older people react to a diagnosis of HIV/AIDS?

Some evidence indicates that the elderly may have different reactions to a diagnosis of HIV compared with younger adults. Following are some of the responses from older adults when asked how they reacted:

- I was glad that I had already had the opportunity for a full life and to see my children grow into adults.

• I was surprised to have HIV, but when you get older you expect to get something like cancer or diabetes sooner or later.

• I think that when you're older, you can cope with things that are unexpected better than younger people because of all your past experiences.

• It's tough getting HIV when you're older because you already have so many health problems.

Despite age differences, the elderly also share many of the experiences that are typical of persons diagnosed with HIV: the fear of being rejected and stigmatized by their family, friends, and community; anger and guilt for becoming infected with a terminal infectious disease because of risky behavior; and fear of infecting another person with the virus.

BIBLIOGRAPHY

1. Adler W, Baskrar P, Chreat F, et al: HIV infection and aging: Mechanisms to explain the accelerated rate of progression in the older patient. Mechan Aging Developt 96:137–155, 1997.
2. Butt A, Dascomb K, DeSalvo, K, et al: Human immunodeficiency virus infection in elderly patients. South Med J 94(4):397–400, 2001.
3. Inungu J, Mokotoff E, Kent J: Characteristics of HIV infection in patients fifty years or older in Michigan. AIDS Patient Care STDs 15(11):567–573, 2001.
4. Keller M, Hausdorff J, Kyne L, Wei J: Is age a negative prognostic indicator in HIV infection or AIDS? Aging 11(1):35–38, 1999.
5. Ory M, Mack K: Middle-aged and older people with AIDS. Res Aging 20:653–663, 1998.
6. Stall R, Cantina J: AIDS risk behaviors among late and middle aged elderly Americans. Arch Intern Med 154:57–63, 1994.

IV. Cultures and Subcultures

21. INJECTION DRUG USERS

San Patten, MSc, and Diane Nielsen, RN, BScN

1. How is the subculture of injection drug users defined?

An injection drug user (IDU) administers drugs by injection with a needle and syringe. The term *injection drug user* is used instead of intravenous drug users (IVDUs) to include all people who inject substances, both legal and illegal, intravenously, intramuscularly, or subcutaneously. A major assumption about IDUs is the existence of a pervasive "drug culture" to which all users belong. This supposed "drug culture" is construed as a group of people who share a common geographical area and common needs and concerns and feel some coherence with one another. In other words, it is assumed that drug users belong to a community, as bounded by the drug-using subculture.

2. Discuss the unique characteristics of IDUs as a subculture.

In discussing the concept of a community or subculture of IDUs, it is important to consider that they are clearly an oppressed and stigmatized group. The act of using illicit drugs in itself creates stigma and pushes IDUs away from the mainstream social center. Although using drugs may also produce social cohesion among IDU peers, it does so at the expense of moving drug users away from the mainstream.[7] Secondly, IDUs who belong to a racial (such as Aboriginal) or sexual minority (such as men who have sex with men or sex trade workers) experience even greater stigmatization. Lastly, poverty pushes people even further to the margins of society. The compounded stigma of drug use, racial or sexual minority, and poverty can reduce the resources available to IDUs.

IDUs have been described as belonging to a "culture of survival."[7] The social organization of IDU subculture is driven by economic deprivation and the common bond of being outcast by society. They are a disenfranchised group—outside mainstream society without access to services because of their lack of conformity to social norms and because of societal prejudice and discrimination. These factors create the need to share resources, including the purchase and sharing of drugs and injection equipment as well as food, shelter, recreation, and other necessities of life. Although IDUs often compete for drugs, money, and even injection equipment, patterns of mutual support are also common. The common bond of being outcast and economically deprived explains much of the violence against the community, society, and each other. When access to food, shelter, recreation, and the other necessities of life is denied to a disenfranchised population, the result is an extremely unstable and volatile social system. IDUs live with the constant challenges of arrest, unstable housing, and little secure income. HIV/AIDS is not their greatest threat.

Social support is an important function of the IDU subculture. Social support can be seen as the emotional, instrumental, and financial aid obtained from one's social network. Social support has several functions that mutually benefit the members of a cohesive community.[8] Members of the IDU subculture share a sense of belonging or a sharing of experience, information, and ideas through relationships and common objectives. Members of an IDU community can provide assistance to one another, either in the provision of tangible goods (e.g., injection equipment) or task-oriented services (e.g., gathering and disposing of used needles, bringing new ones). Finally, members of a community receive mutual guidance and advice, such as through the delivery and exchange of information about health and/or street news.

3. What drugs are most commonly injected?

The Four Most Commonly Injected Drugs and Related Information

DRUG	CLASS	ACTION	SHORT-TERM EFFECTS	LONG-TERM EFFECTS	WITHDRAWAL SYMPTOMS
Cocaine (blow, coke, white, crack)	CNS stimulant	Onset: 15–30 seconds Duration: 45 minutes	Talkative, excited, loss of appetite, irrational; dilated pupils, elevated heart rate and blood pressure, risk of heart failure, restlessness	Impaired judgment, weight loss, paranoia, hallucinations, impotence, psychological dependence	Insomnia, irritability, depression
Methamphetamine (speed, crank)	CNS stimulant	Onset: within seconds Duration: 8–24 hours	Increased euphoria, hallucinations, loss of appetite, increased energy, restlessness, panic	Malnutrition, weight loss; kidney, lung, and brain damage; stroke; death; violent and aggressive behavior, psychological dependence	Extended troubled sleep, extreme hunger, depression, suicidal ideation
Heroin (smack, H, down, junk)	CNS depressant	Onset: within few minutes Duration: 6–8 hours	Initial euphoria, constricted pupils, decreased heart rate, irregular blood pressure, detachment from pain	Weight loss, impotence; heart, liver, and brain damage; physical and psychological dependence	Convulsions, anxiety, diarrhea, abdominal cramps, runny nose, yawning
Morphine (down, mojo)	CNS depressant	Onset: within few minutes Duration: 6–8 hours	Initial euphoria, constricted pupils, decreased heart rate, irregular blood pressure, detachment from pain	Weight loss; impotence; heart, liver, and brain damage; physical and psychological dependence	Convulsions, anxiety, diarrhea, abdominal cramps, runny nose, yawning

CNS = central nervous system.
Adapted from Walton SC: First response guide to street drugs. Burnand Holding Co. 1: 5–8, 22–24, 44–49, 2001.

4. What is meant by the social context of injection drug use?

Social context refers to "the collective features of the social and physical environments that define the social and behavioral characteristics of and settings for injection drug use and risk for HIV infection in a particular neighborhood or social grouping."[10] Social context includes social forces such as interpersonal relations, peer influences (either constructive or destructive), cultural norms, etiquette, social situations, and social settings. It is also important to specify that social interactions and social situations do not necessarily mean friendly or happy relations. Conflict and confrontation are integral parts of social context and exert substantial influence on shaping the social environments within which injection drug use occurs. It is important to consider the nature and role of social contexts of various groups of IDUs because the social networks through which they buy and sell illicit drugs are the same networks through which HIV may be transmitted.

IDUs' drugs of choice are most relevant to the social context within which they practice injection drug use. Other important factors include the following:
- Duration and frequency of drug use
- Physiologic and psychoactive effects
- Cravings that accompany drug addiction
- Stresses of drug dealing
- Variable quality of street drugs
- Possibility of overdose
- Feelings of paranoia
- HIV or hepatitis serostatus

5. How do different social contexts of drug use increase HIV risk?

HIV risk behaviors among IDUs are inextricably intertwined with psychosocial factors. Because HIV infection is acquired almost exclusively in specific behavioral contexts, it follows that we should conceptualize HIV risk in interpersonal and social contexts. HIV prevention initiatives for IDUs should take into account interpersonal relationships as a key variable, paying attention to their duration, behavioral norms, level of commitment, emotional and material connectedness, and level of dependency.[10]

Sharing of drug paraphernalia is affected significantly by peer group influences. Social circumstances and lifestyle factors are more important aspects of needle sharing than individual choice and motivations. Peer groups have a strong impact on needle-sharing behaviors and attitudes around sharing needles and other injection equipment.

6. How is the sex trade linked to injection drug use?

Many IDUs support their drug addiction through the sex trade. Sex trade workers are limited in their ability to prevent HIV infection through simple lack of needle availability while working on the stroll and having to inject in settings such as public washrooms, outdoors, cars, or shooting galleries. Furthermore, there is competition with other prostitutes for clients who are willing to pay higher rates for condomless sex. Many sex trade workers report that they are often high while working on the streets, which limits their ability to make healthy choices. Some sex trade workers engage in "fixing dates," including transactions of sex for drugs or encounters in which the sex trade worker shoots up with the client.

7. What are shooting galleries? How do they increase HIV risk?

The shooting gallery is particularly challenging with respect to HIV prevention. Shooting galleries are apartments or houses where IDUs congregate to buy and inject drugs, particularly cocaine. Shooting galleries can be as impermanent as a hotel room that a dealer uses as he moves from place to place. Shooting galleries are important social settings in the lives of many cocaine users because they are a well-known and fairly quick source of cocaine. Shooting galleries are nodes in an informal social network where members of various social groupings of IDUs gather to purchase and inject drugs. Shooting galleries are an important element in the social networks of IDUs not only because they provide a relatively safe place to inject drugs in terms of hiding from the police as well as access to needles and syringes, but also because they offer an arena for socialization among fellow IDUs and a degree of protection in case of overdose. However, the shooting gallery also presents many situational factors that create higher risk for HIV infection. Cocaine use alone is a risk factor for HIV transmission through needle sharing because of the higher frequency of injecting when people use cocaine. Cocaine users often binge on cocaine, injecting every 15–20 minutes to maintain their high, making it difficult to ensure that a clean needle is used every time. There is also an association between cocaine use and high-risk sexual activities due to its aphrodisiac effects.

There may be a wide variety of people in a shooting gallery at any one time—some who seem apathetic about risk reduction and others who are quite conscious of the risks of disease transmission. Some shooting gallery owners play an important HIV prevention role by providing a supply of needles, bleach, and disposal containers to their customers. There is more opportunity for needle sharing in shooting galleries, simply by virtue of the higher concentration of people under one roof. The potential for HIV or hepatitis transmission is very high since needle sharing is not confined to a cohesive social circle but is diffused among many people (up to 50) who may be strangers to one another. The poor lighting and generally unhygienic conditions make it more likely that injection practices will be unsafe, resulting in poor vein care or infections.

8. What role do drug dealers play in HIV risk?

The social context around drug dealers is also important to consider with respect to HIV risk practices. A drug dealer working out of a shooting gallery may advance his drug business by providing an on-site needle supply. By providing needles to his customers, he ensures that the IDUs will stay around to buy his drugs until their money runs out. However, dealers may be reluctant to provide needles to their customers for fear of turning their home into a shooting gallery. Some dealers may not provide needles for free but charge customers for each new syringe. Selling needles is another way for other dealers to make a profit from IDUs. Dealers may allow only a small circle of contacts to purchase their drugs directly from their homes. Needle sharing is limited in such settings for the following reasons:

- IDUs bring their own needles to the house because of the variance in preferred size of syringe barrels.
- IDUs may prefer to inject privately in separate rooms so that their injection equipment is kept separate.
- Even if the people in the dealer's house share needles, their tight social circle of four or five people is not likely to share outside the group; thus, any blood-borne disease such as HIV or hepatitis will be contained within that group.

Unlike shooting gallery settings, the overlap of friendship groupings in sharing situations is less likely to occur in a dealer's house. Without the mixing of blood from members of large numbers of social or friendship groups of IDUs, there is a less efficient means of viral transmission.[10]

9. How does drug use initiation time affect HIV risk?

Several opportunities for risk assumption behaviors exist during the initiation of an inexperienced IDU. The initiate is probably unwise about the safe dosages of the drug, opening opportunity for overdose.The initiate is also unlikely to carry his or her own sterile syringe and is at the mercy of the experienced IDU to supply sterile injection equipment. The experienced IDU may try to convince the initiate not to be concerned about HIV or hepatitis transmission. The power dynamic between the experienced IDU and the initiate is such that the initiate will have to concede to the conditions set by the experienced IDU. For some IDUs, their first experience is pleasant, but for others it is frightening and hazy. IDUs may not be able to inject themselves when they first start using injection drugs and thus rely on other more experienced IDUs to inject for them. Even if IDUs need assistance with the injection procedure, they should ensure that they know precisely the amount and strength of the drug and the source of the syringe. One of the important harm reduction messages as stated by IDUs is: "Never let somebody else prepare your hit for you."

People who are interested in experimenting with injection drugs are likely to try with or without the assistance of a knowledgeable and experienced IDU. New injectors are less likely than more experienced IDUs to have salient knowledge about drug-related HIV or hepatitis transmission or to attempt risk reduction.[8] From a risk reduction viewpoint, new initiates should be encouraged to seek the assistance of a veteran IDU so that they can be taught proper injection techniques, safe needle handling, and safe dosages. An IDU who is asked by an inexperienced initiate may assist the initiate with HIV prevention by teaching safer injection behaviors.

10. How is injection drug use related to sexual risk behavior?

Injection drug use and sexual risk behavior are linked through several mechanisms:(1) the aphrodisiac effect of cocaine on libido, (2) the exchange of sex for money or drugs, and (3) the effect of mood-altering substances that can impede healthy sexual behavior choices. Addiction to an illicit drug can be expensive, and one common means (particularly for female IDUs) of generating adequate income is the sex trade. For female IDUs, the sex trade offers a quick way to make enough money to support a drug addiction without requiring them to enter the work force of mainstream society. The link between injection drug use and the sex trade is reciprocal because, while prostitution may be initiated by the need for money to finance a drug addiction, the relatively high levels of income generated by prostitution may encourage higher levels of drug use.

Sex trade workers have been identified as a risk group whose lifestyle makes them both particularly vulnerable to infection and a potential conduit of HIV, sexually transmitted diseases (STDs), and hepatitis to the broader community. Drug-injecting sex trade workers are at high risk of contracting STDs, hepatitis, and HIV because of the combination of injection and sexual behaviors. They not only engage in sexual activity with multiple partners whose health status is unknown; they also place themselves at risk if they agree to provide unsafe sexual practices in exchange for their drugs. Women who trade sex for money and/or drugs are less likely to use new needles on a consistent basis or to clean old needles and are more likely to share needles with others compared with women who support themselves by other means.[11]

For many sex trade workers, there is a vicious circle between prostitution and injection drug use: "I have to be high to sell myself, but I have to sell myself to get high."[8] Some prostitutes state that they definitely require a fix of their drug of choice before they are able to turn tricks. The drug high allows them some level of cognitive shielding from the shame and degradation of prostituting themselves or "calm[s] their nerves."[8] Some sex trade workers disclosed that at times they were so high on alcohol and other drugs that they actually blacked out. The next day they could not recall any of the events of the previous night while working on the stroll. Such a high level of impairment places the prostitutes in situations in which they are more likely to adopt risk assumption behaviors and less able to make wise risk reduction choices with respect to both sexual and injecting activities.

Some men who purchase sex (johns) offer higher rates of payment for condomless dates. The more lucrative condomless dates may attract women whose financial needs are high because of their own or their partner's drug habit; therefore, such women are likely to agree more quickly to the absence of a condom.[8] Prostitutes who are more economically dependent on prostitution and perceive less control over the sex trade encounter are more likely to engage in risk assumption behavior.[11]

Many prostitutes go to shooting galleries or dope houses (buildings where drugs are sold and injected) between dates to maintain the high that they need to do their work and to spend the money that they just earned. In most urban centers, the shooting galleries are in close proximity to the main "hooker strolls" so that, as one needle exchange nurse explained, "Girls can go out and get $20 for a blow-job and then into the dope house for a hit of coke, over and over again several times a night."[8]

11. Describe the crisis lifestyle of injection drug use.

IDUs have day-to-day priorities that revolve around their drug addiction. IDUs' first priority is drugs: their quality, their availability, and the money to purchase them. Their addiction leads to obsessive thoughts, compulsive urges, and drug-seeking behavior. Their entire waking hours focus on obtaining and using drugs. Drug cravings and withdrawal symptoms make IDUs unable to endure long waiting periods in medical clinics, social service agencies, or emergency departments. The availability and quality of drugs determine how IDUs will feel each day. With drugs, IDUs can avoid pain and feelings of withdrawal; without them they feel ill and are unable to cope with daily demands. The realities of poverty, unstable housing, and the lack of available resources for daily living result in extended periods of crisis. Other conditions, such as irregular sleeping, poor hygiene, high stress, and poor nutrition, exacerbate the harms of high drug use and further compromise the immune system. IDUs miss health or social service appointments and forget medications, resulting in physical and psychological consequences. They become careless, and the need for the drug becomes stronger than the need for safety. Illicit drug use can involve illegal activity, and IDUs may resort to criminal activity to support their habit. IDUs are often reluctant to reveal their identity because they fear the consequences of outstanding warrants, drug charges, or prostitution charges. Dissatisfaction with and fear or distrust of medical institutions have additional negative effects on IDUs' health. Social isolation becomes the only safe means to ensure survival, and social support may be nonexistent.

12. How are HIV and other blood-borne pathogens transmitted through injection drug use?

One of the primary modes for HIV transmission through intravenous drug injecting is the use of HIV-contaminated syringes, needles, vials, spoons, and other injection equipment. Much of the harm related to injection drug use results from a combination of limited needle availability, poor hygiene surrounding self-injection, and inadequate injection technique. Injecting with dull needles (those that have been used several times) produces larger punctures than necessary, causing skin, tissue, and venous scarring in regular or frequent injectors. Repeated use of damaged sites and improper injection technique may result in abscesses, ulceration, venous scarring, and circulatory damage when veins clog (thrombose) or collapse.

Unsterile skin, syringes, needles, and other paraphernalia can introduce a variety of infectious agents. Contracting HIV or viral hepatitis through using injection equipment with traces of someone else's blood is not the only risk. Organisms common to the skin surface can contribute to the development of bacterial infections. The water used to prepare drugs for injection may provide another source of bacteria, viruses, and other infectious agents. Even skilled IDUs with sterile injection equipment and clean skin cannot prevent injecting the insoluble (and/or harmful) diluents and impurities that most black market drugs contain. Impurities such as talc, cornstarch, quinine, and fibers of cotton or cigarette filters have been implicated in damage to cardiac, skeletal, and smooth muscle; the gastrointestinal tract and kidneys; local tissue destruction; bacterial growth; neurologic lesions; and immunologic abnormalities.

13. Discuss harm reduction in relation to injection drug use.

Harm reduction is a health promotion philosophy that has as its first priority a decrease in the negative consequences of drug use. The harm reduction approach can be contrasted with abstentionism, the dominant policy in North America, which emphasizes elimination of drug use. Harm reduction tries to reduce problems associated with drug use and recognizes that abstinence is not the only acceptable or important goal. Harm reduction involves setting a hierarchy of goals, with the more immediate and realistic ones to be achieved in steps on the way to harm-free use or, if appropriate, abstinence. Consequently, it is an approach characterized by pragmatism. The approach is based on the beliefs that moral condemnation of groups at harm leads to reduction in contact with health services and, therefore, is counterproductive and that the majority of drug users are willing and able to change behavior if the right conditions apply.

Injecting is the most complicated and risky way in which to administer drugs, but its health risks can be significantly reduced by ensuring aseptic injection conditions. Aseptic injection can be simply stated as follows: "New equipment for every hit of drug and hands washed before touching anything or anyone else."[8] Ideally, IDUs should use a new syringe and needle for every injection and are encouraged to stock syringes rather than be caught short. If a clean, unused syringe is unavailable, IDUs are told to clean the syringe with bleach with no guarantee that the cleaning will be 100% effective against HIV or hepatitis C. However, some cleaning is better than none at all. If forced to use an old needle, the best practice is for an IDU to use one of his or her own.

The harm reduction message for HIV prevention among IDUs can be summarized by the following guidelines:
- Get off drugs.
- If you cannot or will not stop using drugs, do not inject them.
- If you inject drugs, use a clean needle every time.
- If you cannot use a clean needle every time, re-use your own needles and do not share with someone else.
- If you have to share needles, at least clean the needles with bleach.[2]

Safer injection also includes good vein care techniques, such as rotating injection sites, using a tourniquet that is easy to release before injecting the drug, and applying pressure to the injection site immediately after the "hit" (injection) until the bleeding stops. IDUs are also encouraged to prevent abscesses, septicemia, and endocarditis by cleaning the injection site with an alcohol swab and using only sterile water to prepare their hit. IDUs should also avoid injecting dirty hits (e.g., hits containing dirt, hairs, fibers) by using a clean spoon and a new filter every time. IDUs can take four main measures to ensure safer injecting:
- Not sharing injection equipment (including needles, syringes, water, spoons, filters, or tourniquets)
- Keeping the procedure aseptic by swabbing spoon, injection site, and fingers with alcohol beforehand
- Cleaning after injections by flushing the syringe to remove all traces of blood, making bleaching easier, if necessary
- Safely disposing of equipment by recapping the needle, placing it in a hard, rigid-walled container, and returning the container to the local needle exchange program

While neither condoning nor condemning drug use, the harm reduction model accepts that drug use continues to occur and that many initiatives can be undertaken to minimize the harm to all involved. This approach does not exclude abstinence as an eventual goal, if the user decides to pursue it. However, the focus is on minimizing the harmful outcomes associated with drug use. Examples of harm reduction initiatives include provision of needle exchange, condoms, information about safe-injecting practices, and safe-injecting rooms or shelters.

14. What are the arguments in favor of needle exchange?

Drug use occurs along a continuum, ranging from minimal to extreme risk. IDUs cannot be forced or convinced to stop using drugs until they feel ready and are able to do so, but the risk associated with drug use can be reduced. IDUs do not readily access conventional health care settings and resources because of their crisis lifestyle and past unfavorable experiences with institutions. Needle exchange programs (NEPs) are a simple, inexpensive way of providing harm reduction tools and services to the IDU population in their own community setting and in an accepting, nonjudgmental manner. The goal of NEPs is the reduction or elimination of a constellation of harms that accompany addiction to drugs and injection drug use. NEPs acknowledge that IDUs are addicted to drugs and that society cares enough about their health to make their drug use as safe as possible, at least until they are ready to discontinue drug use. NEPs approach this high-risk population by offering a range of services and support systems. Many programs go beyond the simple exchange of needles, employing health care professionals to provide health promotion strategies such as HIV and hepatitis testing, immunization, counseling, and reinforcement of prevention messages. NEPs are often the first point of service provision and contact in developing a positive, trusting relationship with drug users. Numerous studies have concluded that NEPs do not increase the use of drugs and can actually reduce the number of HIV infections. Programs that are linked closely with other health or social service agencies can assist users in breaking the cycle of their addiction.

15. What are some arguments against needle exchange?

Some people within the traditional health care and law enforcement systems argue that by supplying clean needles to IDUs, we are enabling them to continue their injection behaviors. In addition, provision of clean needles and other resources in their own settings may bring IDUs together to share resources and thus result in risky behaviors, ultimately increasing the risk for HIV and hepatitis infection. When needles are supplied to IDUs without adequate disposal systems, the needles may be left in the community, putting others at risk. People with health conditions requiring needles for injection (such as diabetes) feel that they could also benefit from free supplies.

16. Why are rates of HIV infection higher among the prison population?

The legal aspects of drug use and their intersection with HIV/AIDS have created an emergency situation in prisons. Many IDUs spend time in prison settings, either directly because of drug convictions or indirectly because of other criminal convictions related to drug use. It is a fact of life that inmates will continue to engage in high-risk behaviors. Unfortunately, administrative responses within correctional services aimed at preventing the spread of HIV have thus far been limited. With the majority of prisoners moving back to the community once their jail terms have been completed, the seriousness of this issue for all members of society cannot be ignored.

Despite the sustained efforts of prison systems to prevent the entry of drugs into prisons, the reality is that drugs can and do enter. A number of studies have provided evidence of the extent of injection and other drug use in prisons.[5] Many prisoners crave some form of drugs. Many of them are in prison because of offenses committed to meet the demands of their drug addiction. Injection drug use is prevalent in prisons, and the scarcity of needles often leads to needle sharing. Drugs are part of prison culture and reality; for inmates addicted to injection drugs, imprisonment increases the risk of contracting HIV infection because of unsafe injection practices within the prisons. Furthermore, some IDUs actually start to inject while in prison.

Unsafe sexual practices in prisons also contribute to the higher rates of HIV infection among inmates. Homosexual encounters are a part of the reality of prison life, and without the confidential and open provision of condoms inmates will engage in unprotected sex (see Chapter 23 for a more detailed discussion).

17. What myths influence society's attitudes toward injection drug use?

Myth: IDUs are less valuable citizens and contribute less to society.

Truth: IDUs do not live in a vacuum. They are members of the community and, both during and after the periods of their lives that involve the injection of drugs, form intimate partnerships and have children. Many IDUs are employed and valuable members of society. They have a secure income, housing, and support network. A portion of their income may be used to support their addiction, but they are still able to function as productive members of society.

Myth: IDUs are criminals unable to overcome their addiction because of moral failure.

Truth: IDUs come from all walks of life, and many have not been incarcerated. Their addiction may be due to a legitimate medical condition that was not given adequate treatment. At the most basic level, attitudes towards IDUs living with HIV or AIDS must be addressed as a first step in the destigmatization and normalization process. A starting point is education of the public and professionals that leads to increased awareness of injection drug use as a health rather than a criminal issue. We need to build awareness, recognition, and acceptance in the justice system and in law enforcement that addiction is better dealt with as a health and social issue than as a criminal one.

Myth: Becoming addicted is the IDU's own fault.

Truth: Initially a person may use a drug for its pleasurable or analgesic effects. Prolonged use can cause changes in the brain that take the person from a voluntary state of drug use to compulsive drug-seeking behavior.

Myth: IDUs do not want to change their behavior and do not respond well to education and treatment intervention.

Truth: Compulsions are often driven by the need to avoid side effects and withdrawal symptoms. Once use of a drug is decreased or terminated, cramps, vomiting, diarrhea or depression may result. IDUs may not be able to tolerate the physical or psychological withdrawal symptoms without adequate treatment or support. Thus they may return to drug use.

Myth: Needle exchange programs encourage drug users to continue or start injecting drugs.

Truth: People who are addicted to a substance will find a way to inject the drug, regardless of whether they have access to a safe supply of injection equipment. NEPs provide a means for IDUs to obtain harm reduction tools for prevention of HIV and hepatitis C infection but do not entice people to begin injection drug use. Evidence shows the following:
- NEPs are effective in reducing the spread of HIV.
- NEPs do not increase the number of IDUs or lower the age of initiation into injection drug use.
- NEPs do not increase the number of needles discarded in a community or change the locations where needles are disposed.[4]

18. What dos and don'ts are important in working with IDUs?

Dos
- Recognize your own biases and how they can affect interaction with clients.
- Respect all clients.
- React without judgment and accept the client's decisions and choices.
- Be patient with yourself and your clients.
- Be supportive despite relapse.
- Regard clients as separate from the drug. IDUs are persons who react from a drug.
- Listen to clients' stories; not all answers are in a textbook.
- Encourage safe drug use and safe sex practices.

Don'ts
- Do not expect abstinence until the user is ready to quit.
- Do not talk down to clients. They are experts in their field and have extensive knowledge that they can share with you.
- Do not reject clients or act superior for having made different choices.

19. What is the LIGHT model of care? How can it be used to help HIV-positive IDUs reach optimal health?

The LIGHT model[1] uses intervention to improve clients' self-esteem, leading them to take a greater interest in their health care needs. Through personalized care and perception of individual needs, IDUs have a greater chance of reaching their full potential. Bonding is the first step in the process. Nurses must be alert for opportunities to develop trust and rapport with the clients. The next step involves identifying clients' state of well-being and the barriers that prevent them from improving their health situation. Their concerns and talents should be recognized at this time. Once they identify their talents, they are more likely to believe that they are worthy of care. The last step encourages the clients to take action through teaching new skills, providing support, and promoting new talents. Through personalized nursing intervention clients are assisted with the initial steps in addressing their concerns, which then encourages them to repeat the process independently with future issues and difficulties.

The LIGHT Model

FACETS OF THE PROCESS	ROLE OF NURSES AND CAREGIVERS	ROLE OF CLIENT
Bond	Love the client Intend to help Give care gently	Love yourself Identify a concern Give yourself a goal
Assess well-being and identify barriers	Help client improve well-being	Have confidence and help yourself
Teach the LIGHT model	Teach a healing process and help the client plan the first step to deliberate pattern change	Take positive action

From Andersen MD, Smereck GAD, Hockman EM, et al: Nurses decrease barriers to health care by "hyperlinking" multiple-diagnosed women living with HIV/AIDS into care. J Assoc Nurses AIDS Care 10(2): 55–65, 1999.

20. Discuss the special needs of HIV-positive IDUs.

Addressing the multiple difficulties in seeking appropriate, accessible treatment for a substance use problem can be overwhelming, as it can also be for HIV infection. Barriers to accessing care when both conditions are present—particularly if other issues, such as mental illness, are also involved—can seem insurmountable. People with these conditions may have to confront discriminatory and/or uninformed attitudes on the part of treatment providers. In addition, availability of appropriate treatment sites is frequently limited. Decision-making about the best treatment approach is often taken out of the hands of the client for fear, on the part of the health care providers, that an injection drug user will not comply with treatment regimens. Pain may not be well-managed by physicians unwilling to prescribe adequate medication to patients with a history of substance use, fearing the risk of overdose or supporting the addiction.

IDUs living with HIV must be recognized as people who suffer in a myriad of ways and need the best possible interventions, tailored to their unique situations. They retain all of the rights of every other citizen and, therefore, must be given equal access to a continuum of services as well as the dignity of making their own decisions. If lack of compliance with a drug treatment is feared, patients must be supported to ensure adherence, just as any other patient is, whether diagnosed with diabetes, epilepsy, or another condition. Bias against treating IDUs is unjustified and unacceptable.[3]

21. How can health promotion strategies be coordinated to help IDUs make healthier lifestyle choices?

Health care providers must have a contextual understanding of drug injection, the culture of drug use, and the stages and form of addiction among different subgroups of drug users.[8] Such understanding allows health practitioners and programmers to design and implement risk reduction interventions that will be accepted within, and integrated into, current social networks. Risk practices, such as needle sharing, are shaped by social interactions and social norms. The entire process of purchasing, pooling, preparing, and injecting drugs occurs within a social context of deeply engrained rituals. It follows that interventions targeted to reduce the risk of injection drug use also must be shaped by social interactions and social norms. For example, interventions for women who trade sex for money or drugs should focus on supplying sterile injection equipment to prostitutes while they are working, culturally sensitive counseling about the risks of unprotected sex, and encouraging and making accessible drug treatment and alternate sources of employment to end the vicious circle of prostitution and drug addiction.

For interventions with IDUs to be successful, health and social service providers must discover ways to work together. All health and social service partners need to be involved in a client-centered, integrated service delivery approach to facilitate higher-quality, comprehensive, consistent, and cost-effective care. The sharing of skills, experience, and ideas is more likely to achieve a reduction in HIV risk behavior and addiction in IDUs. IDUs need to be made aware of the services that are available to them, and these services should be easily accessible. The services must be brought into the settings where IDUs gather—homes, parks, shooting galleries, and hotels. Offering the clients as many services as possible in one location encourages their return to the agency. Providing addiction counseling, health care, and needle exchange at one location effectively increases the quality of care that IDUs receive.[6]

Key service providers who must collaborate to provide comprehensive services to IDUs include but are not limited to the following:

• Substance use programs and facilities
• Harm reduction programs
• HIV treatment facilities and hospices
• Community-based AIDS service organizations
• Departments or ministries of health, justice, and social services
• Regional health authorities
• Public health centers
• Outreach programs
• Homeless agencies
• Pharmaceutical companies

In order to access services, IDUs need to feel comfortable with the staff in the organization. A nonjudgmental, sensitive approach that recognizes their need for confidentiality is more likely to achieve positive results in making healthier choices. Staff should be trained to overcome their own biases and social stigmas to provide effective interventions for disease prevention and health promotion.

According to HIV prevention literature, the most effective means to address prevention of HIV transmission is through behavior change—and this goal can be achieved only through effective education strategies and community mobilization. Effective prevention programs must be community-based and culturally appropriate, but the challenge is in defining the "community" and the "culture." Therefore, health professionals should be working toward peer-based programs that allow IDUs to become empowered to define, analyze, and act upon their own problems.

BIBLIOGRAPHY

1. Andersen MD, Smereck GAD, Hockman EM, et al: Nurses decrease barriers to health care by "hyper-linking" multiple-diagnosed women living with HIV/AIDS into care. J Assoc Nurses AIDS Care 10(2):55–65, 1999.
2. Calgary Health Region: Creating a Healthy Community for Women Living with HIV, Training and Resource Manual for Care Providers. Calgary, Alberta, Calgary Health Region, 2001.
3. Canadian Centre on Substance Abuse and Canadian Public Health Association: HIV, AIDS and Injection Drug Use: A National Action Plan. Ottawa, Ontario, Canadian Centre on Substance Abuse and Canadian Public Health Association, 1997.
4. Canadian HIV/AIDS Legal Network: Injection Drug Use and HIV/AIDS: Legal and Ethical Issues. Montreal, Quebec, Canadian HIV/AIDS Legal Network, 1999.

5. Gore S, Birg G: HIV, hepatitis and drugs epidemiology in prisons. In Shewan D, Davies JB (eds): Drug Use and Prisons: An International Perspective. Amsterdam, Harwood Academic, 1999.

6. Health Canada: HIV/AIDS Epi Update: HIV/AIDS Among Injection Drug Users in Canada. Ottawa, Ontario, Health Canada, 2001.

7. Moore LD, Wenger LD: The social context of needle exchange and user self-organization in San Francisco: Possibilities and pitfalls. Drug Issues 25(3): 583–598, 1995.

8. Patten S: The Social Context of HIV Risk Assumption and Risk Reduction Strategies Employed by Injection Drug Users. Calgary, Alberta, University of Calgary Thesis, 1999.

9. Walton SC: First response guide to street drugs. Burnand Holding Co. 1: 5–8, 22–24, 44–49, 2001.

10. Watters JK: Impact of HIV risk and infection and the role of prevention services. J Substance Abuse Treat 13(5): 375–385, 1996.

11. Wermuth L, Ham J, Robbins RL: Women don't wear condoms: AIDS risk among sexual partners of IV drug users. In Huber J, Schneider BE (eds): The Social Context of AIDS. London, Sage Publications, 1992.

22. CULTURALLY COMPETENT CARE

Donna M. Gallagher, RNCS, MS, ANP, FAAN

Cultural competence is the ability of a person to perform professional tasks effectively for all of the different racial, ethnic, linguistic, and cultural groups accessing services. Minority populations have been disproportionately affected by the HIV/AIDS epidemic since the beginning. As early as 1982, almost one-fifth of the initially reported cases were among African-Americans, who at that time represented only 12% of the United States population.[1] In 2002, minority populations represent over one-half of the HIV/AIDS cases, with steady increases expected in the future. Nurses serve an essential and unique role in the delivery of HIV/AIDS prevention, care, and treatment programs. When nurses understand the importance of providing culturally competent care for persons living with HIV who are minorities, a safe environment develops and leads to both high-quality care and increased access.

1. What should nurses know about minority health beliefs?

First, historical circumstances have created a context for understanding the responses of minority communities to the health care system and vice versa. The following are examples of activities that have affected the relationship between the two.

Tuskegee Syphilis Study

From 1932 through 1972, under the auspices of the United States Public Health Service (USPHS), researchers subjected African-American men in rural Alabama to an experiment on the effects of untreated syphilis. Researchers withheld treatment and forbade the men from seeking help elsewhere, even though penicillin became available in 1940. The experiment was stopped in 1972—only after it came to public attention. Since the closure of the study, the events have become much more than an isolated event in history. We are reminded of the racism in science and the potential misuse of power by those in government as well as medicine toward vulnerable people.[8]

Los Angeles Vaccine Study

In 1989 the Centers for Disease Control (CDC), Kaiser Permanente, and Johns Hopkins University conducted a study of 1,500 children in West and East Los Angeles. The children were given an experimental measles vaccine as part of a government-sponsored trial. Most subjects were Latino or African-American. Parents were not told that their children were part of an unlicensed drug experiment. This study was stopped after 2 years when questions were raised about the vaccine's relationship to an increased death rate among female infants.[2]

In addition, two significant events occurred early in the HIV/AIDS epidemic:

- The origin of AIDS was thought to be tied to Africa. This theory led to an increase in discrimination against African Americans.
- Early high-risk groups included Haitians. The CDC removed Haitians from the list in 1985, but the damage was already done. It was not until mid 1980 that blood banks removed Haitians from a list of "potential carriers."[5]

Understanding these events and their impact on minorities, particularly community mistrust of the health care system, better equips nurses to respond appropriately to the needs of minority persons with HIV. Nurses should be careful to ask their patients about their usual patterns of accessing health care and what their preferences are (e.g., clinic-based services, hospital emergency department, healer, male/female, person of color).

2. Why is it important to understand the social situation in which the patient lives and the community norms related to HIV?

Twenty years into the HIV epidemic, many communities still subscribe to mistaken ideas: HIV is contagious, HIV is a punishment from God, or HIV is a gay disease or a disease of drug addicts and prostitutes. Many still believe that people with HIV should be isolated and not allowed in public.

The nurse and patient should discuss who the patient has told about his or her HIV status and whether it is permissible to talk about it in front of other family members. Ask the patient to describe how his or her family and community have reacted and whether he or she has concerns about safety if the information is made public. This information becomes critically important in home care settings when a nurse enters the patient's surroundings. We are always guests in patients' homes and must abide by their rules to preserve trust in the relationship.

3. How do we integrate the role of cultural healing and complementary therapies in the minority setting?

Each culture has traditions and beliefs that are passed on from generation to generation. Home remedies, ethnic medicine, and healers have been part of history throughout the ages. In the past ten years these therapies have gained more respect in Western medicine and are frequently incorporated into a patient's care. In some cases, insurance companies will even pay for these treatments. A nurse should ask what other types of medicines the patient is taking, including home remedies (e.g., tonics, herbal drinks, Chinese black pills, mistletoe). The nurse should also be aware of traditional medical techniques, such as blood letting, cupping, and potions.

Asking a patient to explain the practice or medication delivers a nonjudgmental message and allows the nurse to obtain critical information. In most cases, little evidence-based practice information is available for tonics and herbs. However, the body of information is increasing as these remedies undergo study as adjuncts to Western medicine. A prescription to add yoga, massage, vitamins, tai chi, and/or other complementary therapies is seen quite regularly in the HIV care plan.

4. How important is the patient's primary language?

The person who sits before you may speak English as the primary language or may identify one of hundreds of other languages as the primary language. When English is not the primary language, an interpreter should be called for the visit. A patient in a stressful situation often hears only a small percentage of the discussion. The percentage is even smaller when the information is not in the patient's primary language. If an interpreter is used, the nurse should make every effort to meet the following goals:

- Meet with the interpreter to review the goals for the session
- Provide an opportunity for the interpreter and patient to meet before the session begins
- Encourage the interpreter to deliver your message verbatim
- Be patient, speak slowly, and use clear, simple language.

Be sure to give written information in English and, whenever possible, in the patient's primary language. The interpreter must agree to maintain the patient's confidentiality. If only English literature is available, ask the interpreter to write important decisions or pieces of information in the primary language.

5. How does culture influence the role of multiple sexual partners and men who have sex with men?

Each culture has its own set of norms regarding sexual partners. These norms differ widely and are not always freely discussed. The norms of a patient's culture may not be the same as our own; therefore, it is important to approach this discussion in a nonjudgmental way.

Consider, for example, a young Latino who has been diagnosed with HIV. She tells you that she had no risks of which she knows and that she is married. She may not want to tell you that some men in the Latin culture have several sexual partners, including other men. The men do not think of themselves as homosexual, and the women understand that other men and women are having sex with their husbands. She is aware that her husband has other sexual partners.

The nurse may start this type of conversation by acknowledging that in many cultures the men have varied sexual experiences. Ask the patient to describe her culture and how she feels about the norms. This may also be a good time to ask her to share any other information about her culture that she thinks will help with her health care. Engaging the patient as your educator facilitates the trust relationship and, hopefully, empowers her to participate in decisions about her care.

6. Who is the decision maker in terms of health care?

It is essential to identify who makes decisions about health care as early as possible in the relationship with a patient. Many cultural rules relate to examination, including who is allowed to speak to a woman about her health and who will make decisions about health. Consider the following examples:

- A young Pakistani woman is in need of an operation to remove her appendix. She has refused to discuss the operation or be examined fully until her husband arrives home from a business trip. He gives permission for her to be examined but insists that he be present for the exam. He signs the operating room consent.
- A middle-aged man from Northern Africa refuses to be examined by a woman and is angry that she makes direct eye contact with him.
- A young woman from Thailand will not lift her eyes when you speak to her and will not make eye contact. This is a sign of respect for a professional who, she feels, is of higher rank than herself.

The nurse who is trying to provide care can be extremely frustrated and ineffective if the time is not taken to understand such cultural norms. When patients refuse interventions, it is often because of cultural conflict. Taking a few minutes to understand the patient's culture will allow the nurse to be an advocate and successful provider.

Many unwritten rules are the cultural norm in a patient's homeland. The fact that he or she is obtaining health care in the U.S. does not imply that native culture was left behind. The nurse who takes the time to explore a patient's culture is more likely to enjoy a positive relationship with the patient—and certainly the nurse will learn a great deal.

7. How is end-of-life care viewed in minority communities?

Every culture has its own view of death and rituals associated with death and dying. The hospice concept is widely recognized in England and the United States as a culturally acceptable way to provide end-of-life care. However, this model has been infrequently used in minority communities. African-American, Haitian, Latino, and several Asian cultures see the care of the elderly and dying as the responsibility of the younger generations.

During the HIV epidemic inpatient hospices were overflowing, and home hospices had waiting lists. As the epidemic shifted to minority communities, hospices began to see empty beds, and as the era of highly active antiretroviral therapy (HAART) was introduced, many hospices closed completely.

Nurses providing end-of-life care for minority patients with HIV need to understand cultural beliefs about dying and what rituals are followed. For example:

- Who is to be at the bedside?
- Who can participate in the intimate care of the dying patient?
- What will happen if the family cannot manage the care at home?
- Is hospice care an option. or is it more culturally acceptable to die in the hospital surrounded by family?
- What rituals should be observed after death? Should the body be left alone for a certain time until the spirit crosses to the other side? Should the body be buried immediately before the next sundown? Should the body be wrapped in herbs and covered with holy oils?

These are some of the many rituals and traditions that may need to be recognized so that family members feel that their loved one is at peace.

8. How can high-quality HIV care be delivered to the homeless?

Providing health care for homeless patients can be both rewarding and challenging. Many providers feel that it is futile to treat homeless patients unless they are hospitalized. Some carry it even further by withholding treatments such as HAART, a highly successful

HIV medication regimen. Although health care for the homeless is delivered primarily in emergency settings, many homeless patients have successfully taken complex medication regimens for diabetes, hypertension, and HIV. Successful strategies to deliver care to the homeless include the following:

- Meet with the homeless patient at the site where he or she spends most of the time.
- Identify where he or she sleeps at night. Does he or she have access to water, bathrooms, and a safe place for medications?
- Create a calendar of meeting times and set some dates with the patient. This is one way to determine whether the patient can reliably meet with you on a weekly basis.
- Determine whether the patient is willing to try a mock adherence trial. (A patient is given candy or placebo pills and is asked to take them as if they were the real drug regimen).
- Ask the patient to identify when and where he or she is most comfortable meeting with you. Some patients get their meals at soup kitchens and have a well-established routine that may facilitate the ability to keep appointments with the nurse.
- If the patient spends time in a shelter, the nurse should meet with the shelter staff to evaluate their willingness to participate in a plan with the patient.

Consistent health care is not the goal for all homeless persons. The nurse can use these strategies and hopefully find success with some homeless patients. As with all patients, we can offer our best opportunities, but the patient must accept the offer. Many homeless patients turn down the offer. The nurse's role in such cases is that of advocate and facilitator; if the patient turns down the offer today, you need to make it again another day. When the patient is ready, he or she will accept the offer, and the nurse will be ready to respond.

Clearly the most important step in evaluating a nurse's cultural competency is self-assessment. The following assessment has been used prior to several cultural competency training sessions as a self-evaluation tool. The nurse who takes a moment to think about the questions and answers will be guided in caring for minority patients with HIV.

Cross- Cultural Encounters: A Comfort Level Guide

Directions: During your professional interactions with people from different cultural backgrounds, you may encounter the following situations. As you read each statement, answer the following question to yourself: How comfortable would you be if you encountered any of these scenarios? Circle the number on the "Comfort Scale" that most clearly resembles your feelings.

1	2	3	4	5
Completely Comfortable	Moderately Comfortable	Ambivalent	Moderately Uncomfortable	Extremely Uncomfortable

1. A patient who does not make "eye contact". _____
2. Coworkers speaking to each other in their primary languages. _____
3. A patient reveals to you that he or she has not been successful with the medical treatment because he or she has been hexed. _____
4. Patients who arrive late for their appointments. _____
5. Interviewing a patient who has a heavy accent. _____
6. Perceptions of illness related to the supernatural and/or spirituality. _____
7. Someone standing too close to you when conversing. _____
8. Beliefs that oral health screening may harm the body. _____
9. Using formal titles to address patients. _____
10. A patient who wishes to have family members present during their exam. _____
11. Patients who rely on home remedies to treat their health problems. _____
12. Having to use an interpreter. _____

From Deoshor Haig and Associates, Cultural Competency Consultants, Providence, RI, with permission.

BIBLIOGRAPHY

1. Centers for Disease Control and Prevention: HIV/AIDS Surveillance Report July 8, 1982.
2. Cimons M: US measles experiment failed to disclose risk. Washington Post A8, June 17, 1996.
3. Cross-Cultural Encounters: A Comfort Level Guide. Deoshor Haig and Associates, Cultural Competency Consultants, Providence, RI.
4. Gardenswartz L, Rowe A: Managing Diversity in Health Care. San Francisco, Jossey-Bass, 1998.
5. Haiti Progress. This Week in Haiti 13(9):24-30, May, 1995.
6. Smith DK, et al: HIV/AIDS among African-Americans: Progress or progression? AIDS 14:1237–1248, 2000.
7. Thomas SB, Quinn SC: The Tuskegee Syphilis Study, 1932 to 1972: Implications for HIV education and AIDS risk education programs in the Black community. Am J Public Health 81:1498–1505, 1991.
8. Tuskegee Syphilis Study Legacy Committee: Final Report. May 20, 1996.
9. United Nations General Assembly: Draft Declaration of the World Conference against Racism, Racial Discrimination, Xenophobia and Related Intolerance. New York, United Nations General Assembly, 2001.

23. HIV/AIDS BEHIND BARS

Pamela J. Dole, EdD, MPH, FNP, ACRN

This chapter explores special considerations for the care of persons with HIV/AIDS behind bars. Nurses have an excellent opportunity to create and implement compassionate care for offenders. Endless opportunities exist for health education and promotion. A brief discussion of the incarceration of disenfranchised populations provides nurses with insight about the prison population.

The faces behind bars have always been disproportionately from minority, poor, vulnerable, and disenfranchised populations. Minority groups have risen significantly over the past decade. Non-Hispanic white offenders account for 41.9% of prison populations; non-Hispanic blacks for 41.3%; Hispanics for 15.1%; and other races (Asians, Pacific Islanders, American Indians, and Alaska Natives) for 1.6%. Male inmates account for 88.6% of local jail populations.[4] Female prisoners have increased by 2-fold over the past two decades and currently account for 6.7% of prisoners.[3,4]

This diverse population is incarcerated in local, state, and federal facilities. Local facilities, which include county or city jails and detention or holding centers, have the highest turnover because length of stay ranges from several hours to several months. State prisons generally house inmates for more than 1 year and for more serious offenses. Federal prisons or penitentiaries incarcerate persons who committed offenses against the U.S. government. Transitional programs, such as work camps, work release, and court programs, incorporate employment generally off the grounds of correctional facilities during the day; inmates return to the correctional facility at night and during the weekend. Forensic psychiatric institutions house court-mandated persons with severe mental illness who have committed offenses against the state or federal government. During incarceration all rights are lost except for humanitarian treatment, including health care.

1. What is the prevalence rate of HIV/AIDS infection among incarcerated people?

HIV/AIDS infection is 7 times higher in prisoners than in the general population. HIV infection rates in correctional facilities continue to rise and vary from location to location. Local jails often have the highest rates. Within state correctional facilities the HIV infection rates are as follows: 7.5 % in the Northeast, 2 % in the South, 1.1 % in the Midwest, and 0.8 % in the West. New York state prisons house half of all HIV cases behind bars in the Northeast.[13] Within the federal penitentiaries the HIV infection rate is 5%.

The rates of HIV infection among incarcerated women are double those of men in the same geographic area. The Northeast has the highest rates of HIV infection among incarcerated women. In New York state prisons, 29% of women and 14% of men are HIV-infected (Alexis Lang, MD, personal communication, 2002).

The majority of women learn their HIV status while incarcerated or during pregnancy. Inadequate nursing and medical histories fail to assess risk factors for HIV.[13] Lack of prevention directed specifically at women has contributed to steadily rising HIV/AIDS transmission rates over the past two decades.[14] The response to rising HIV rates among women was to initiate mandatory HIV testing for pregnant women in New York and Connecticut. This controversial policy raises ethical human rights concerns. Other women are not tested because they do not access health care.

2. What are the primary reasons that people with HIV/AIDS are incarcerated?

Drug-related offenses are the primary reason for incarceration. The majority of drug-related offenders were using drugs within the 30 days before incarceration, and 75% have a history of substance abuse, including alcoholism. Approximately 75% of current prison populations are not violent offenders. Female offenses include violent crimes (25–33%), and drug-related offenses such as loitering, possession, or burglary account for 40–70% of the nonviolent crimes. Males commit more violent crimes (approximately 40% of offenders).

3. How has legislation affected the increase in prison rates?

In 2001 the U.S. incarcerated two million nonviolent prisoners as a direct response to increasingly stringent sentencing laws, which culminated in The Violent Crime Control and Law Enforcement Act of 1994 (refined from the 1987 act). In the 1987 act the United States responded to the frustration of citizens and law enforcement by enacting stiffer prison sentences. This law is commonly called the War on Drug Laws or the Rockefeller Laws. It was strengthened with the 1994 federal crime bill when financial incentives were added to state budgets after certain offenders served 85% of their sentence. Under the state and federal drug laws, crack carries a mandatory prison sentence for first-time possession. Unfortunately, this law has barely affected high-level drug dealers.

4. For which infection are inmates most commonly at risk while incarcerated?

Tuberculosis (TB) remains the single most communicable disease behind bars, where it occurs 5 times more frequently than in the general population.[21,30] The prevalence of TB behind bars is 7–10%, in part because of confined space with overcrowding, poor ventilation, and increased community rates of TB and HIV.[10] Correctional systems have experienced two outbreaks of TB, the first in 1990 and the second in 2000. Multidrug resistant (MDR) TB is also problematic behind bars. The initial outbreak prompted mandatory TB testing in 73% of all correctional facilities with slightly higher rates of mandatory testing in state prisons and lower rates of required testing in jails. Correctional facilities have a responsibility to protect offenders from contracting communicable diseases; after the issues of safety and security, public health is a primary objective.

5. How do security issues affect incarcerated people with HIV/AIDS?

Confinement and security issues are the primary responsibility of prisons. Routines within correctional facilities can inadvertently affect HIV/AIDS medication adherence. Prison administrators and correctional officers (COs) must be educated about the importance of maintaining strict medication adherence with a minimum of missed doses of antiretroviral therapy. COs often possess limited knowledge about HIV/AIDS disease and expressed the most negative attitudes about HIV-infected persons.[17,27] Nurses must remember that COs have no medical knowledge and cannot be expected to monitor offenders' medications.

Prison routines that are the most problematic for medication adherence include transferring offenders for court appearances, health care appointments, refilling medications in a timely manner, lockdowns and searches, and safety transfers to other facilities that occur in the middle of the night with no notice to health care professionals and without medications. Unfortunately, on arrival at the second institution a transferred inmate has no medications and must wait to see a physician. After seeing the health care provider, the offender often waits from 1–2 weeks to receive the medications, because most facilities provide medication through contracts with pharmaceutical companies.

Electronic records have helped to create continuity of health care for offenders frequently transferred to other facilities for security reasons. Approximately 18–20 state and federal institutions have electronic medical records that can easily follow offenders, thereby reducing missed medications, repeated procedures and laboratory tests, and facilitating health care provider visits.

6. Are HIV/AIDS offenders treated differently from other inmates?

Offenders fear being stigmatized if their HIV/AIDS status is known. Confidentiality is difficult to maintain in any closed system. Often confidentiality is breached unintentionally when clients are observed in medication lines or at the HIV specialist clinic (either within or outside the prison) or when they are assigned to special housing.

Correctional facilities protect confidentiality in a number of ways. In most institutions only health care personnel have access to medical information and HIV status of offenders. Administrators have access to this information, on an as-needed basis, to operate facilities. Correctional officers do not have access to medical information, although they often learn it from other offenders. Maintaining medication lines that are sufficiently spaced to allow individual privacy is another example of how institutions can protect confidentiality.

In states such as Alabama, Mississippi, Georgia, and South Carolina, HIV/AIDS populations are housed in one facility. This practice has become a highly debated human rights issue. Offenders complain that they are being stigmatized. Prison officials state that separate housing is the only way that they can provide high-quality health care in a cost-effective manner and reduce HIV transmission. However, aggregate HIV/AIDS housing has been shown to contribute to TB outbreaks.[34] Offenders assigned to HIV/AIDS segregated housing are then identified by association. Throughout the past decade prison policy to segregate HIV-infected offenders from the rest of the prison population has been upheld by the U.S. Supreme Court (January 18, 1900 and 2000), which stated that HIV/AIDS segregation did not violate the Rehabilitation Act of 1973.[40] The ruling also denounced the policy as discriminating against offenders who test positive for HIV.

7. Is mandatory HIV testing of offenders the prevailing policy?

Sixteen states have mandatory HIV testing at admission. Some prisons have neither mandatory testing nor optimal voluntary testing; thus, the reported HIV rates are low.

HIV testing is an important component of diagnosis and treatment. Voluntary testing that has the support and confidence of offenders is imperative to a good program. Offenders will use voluntary testing when they trust that the results are confidential and when they believe that good treatment options are available.

Sufficient education and counseling must accompany HIV testing. Both are required to prevent increased anxiety and possible suicide, to allow hope, to replace myths with facts, to decrease denial regarding risk factors, and to create a plan of action that adequately addresses treatment options.

The issue of partner notification must be explored as well. Before the HIV test results are returned, it is important to know whether an offender fears retribution from a partner or family members or has economic concerns that make dealing with this issue sensitive. Women are at increased risk for abandonment and domestic violence when partners have been notified about their risk for HIV transmission.[36] Centerforce provides peer-led HIV educational programs that discuss risk factors for acquiring HIV with women visiting male offenders.[20]

8. Is HIV/AIDS education available in correctional facilities?

Approximately 66% of correctional facilities reported having HIV/AIDS educational programs in 1997. However, few correctional facilities used HIV/AIDS peer education programs (7% prisons, 3% jails, and 3% penitentiaries) to provide information to offenders and to develop skills that can be applied after released.[22] The AIDS Counseling and Education (ACE) program at Bedford Hills, New York, is one of the original models and has been implemented nationally on a limited basis.[1,6,41] New York has expanded the program to the other state prisons under the name Prisoners AIDS Counseling and Education (PACE). In the San Francisco area, Marin AIDs Project (MAP) and Centerforce also provide peer-led HIV/AIDS education. However, the existence of an educational program does not guarantee attendance or utilization by offenders. Comprehensive educational programs include the following elements:

- Orientation
- Peer education
- Community-based prevention and education
- Individual prevention and education, on request
- Written and audiovisual materials
- Prevention and education in prerelease, day reporting, and pretrial populations
- Gender-specific programs at facilities housing women
- Expansion of HIV curriculums to cover other communicable diseases
- Programs and materials in Spanish and English[22] (p. 27)

A number of other factors contribute to successful peer-led programs.[1] Correctional officers must be included in the planning stage to decrease resistance. Applicants must be screened for sincerity and commitment and sufficient incarceration time to contribute significantly to the program. Peer educators should reflect the ethnocultural make-up of the facility. Incentives for peer educators may include earning "good time," job slots, or academic credits. The curriculum should reflect the needs of the inmates. Involvement of outside organizations (e.g., AIDS service organizations, schools of nursing, or public health agencies) as key leaders demonstrates independence from the correctional facility and increases trust for the programs among offenders.

9. What antiretroviral (ART) adherence issues do HIV/AIDS offenders face?

The routine of prison life certainly affects medication adherence (see question 5). The following factors will also affect adherence to ART:

- Relationships between offenders and health care professionals
- Pill burden
- Directly observed therapy (DOT) vs. keep on person (KOP) medications
- Food requirements
- Education
- Denial about disease
- Untreated mental illness
- Low literacy levels

Research has shown that adherence and acceptance of medications depend on three factors: good interpersonal relationships with providers and peers, trust in the health care system, and trust in the medication.[2,23,32,35] On a day-to-day basis, adherence to medications and withholding of medications by correctional staff as a form of punishment are ongoing challenges.

10. What are the advantages and disadvantages of DOT vs. KOP therapy?

Whether to require DOT or to allow KOP or matched self-administered groups is often a matter of prison policy, and each policy has its strengths and weaknesses. A recent Florida study compared HIV viral suppression with DOT and KOP. The findings showed that 85% of the DOT compared with 50% of the KOP group had a viral suppression (plasma HIV RNA) of less than 50 copies/ml at week 48.[15] This study may greatly affect decisions about medication administration and the reintroduction of clinical trials behind bars. Offenders often object to DOT, stating that it labels them as HIV-infected because the number and frequency of doses exceed those of medications for other chronic diseases. Twice daily and daily ART regimens have reduced the frequency of doses but have not always reduced the pill burden.

11. Why are food requirements a major concern?

ART requiring food restrictions may also be difficult behind bars. Institutional food is often nonappealing; as a result, offenders must keep food in their cubicles. Lack of refrigeration limits choices to canned and nonperishable food that are often fatty and salty. Diets seldom represent the basic food groups. Eating only foods kept in the cubicle is not sufficient to maintain weight for HIV-infected offenders suffering from wasting syndrome. Good nutrition is an essential component of health and well-being and is critical for HIV-infected offenders.

12. Discuss the role of mental illness in adherence to medical regimens.

Undiagnosed and/or untreated mental illness is a major factor in nonadherence to medical regimens. Psychiatric disorders contribute to risk-taking behavior and compromise adherence to complicated medical regimes because of inmates' lack of focus and comprehension; paranoia, doubt, and mistrust; fear disproportionate to situation; and decreased motivation and ability for self-care.[5] Approximately one-third to one-half of offenders have some form of mental illness. Most offenders report varying severity of anxiety and depression during incarceration. Ninety percent of incarcerated women suffer from severe anxiety and depression.[28]

Correctional institutions predominately house the poor. A strong link exists among the cycles of violence, poverty (poor access to care), and mental illness, although there is no consensus about the exact interrelationship. A large majority of female offenders (78%) and 30% of male offenders have experienced physical and sexual abuse before incarceration.[8,24] Many women have seen violence in their environment on a daily basis; this factor contributes significantly to post-traumatic stress disorder (PTSD).[19] Men who experience daily violence in the ghettos report lower rates of PTSD. Researchers postulate that the long history of victimization, secondary to power inequities in conjunction with physical and sexual abuse, contributes to the higher rates of PTSD in incarcerated women. The combination of mental illness and PTSD may also contribute to criminal behavior leading to incarceration.[26,31]

Persons with a history of sexual abuse disconnect from self-care or health promoting behavior.[29] This is especially evident in incarcerated people. Examples include refusal of care, including HIV testing or ART treatment. Offenders with PTSD who agree to ART have difficulty with maintaining the regimen. Common scenarios include the following:

- Increased ART side effects
- Increased ambivalence, with frequent stopping and starting
- Increased fears that the medications will not work
- Increased doubt of the ability to care for self, including management of medications
- Increased subconscious sabotage (e.g., running out of medications)
- Decreased ability to negotiate for self needs
- Decreased boundaries

Incarcerated people with histories of mental illness and/or substance abuse often have alienated families and friends before incarceration, leaving them vulnerable behind bars. Social support from the outside contributes to negotiating power behind bars by having extra supplies or commissary money to trade for favors. Impoverished offenders are often subject to coercion to gain "extra necessities."

13. Do HIV-positive offenders receive the same standard of care as the community population even though HIV medications are so expensive?

Incarcerated persons are the only group in the U.S. that has a legal right to medical care. In 1926, the *Spicer v. Williams* Supreme Court case (191 N.C. 487) stated that the public must care for prisoners who, because they are deprived of their liberties, cannot care for themselves. This ruling fell short of recognizing the prisoners' constitutional rights under the Eighth Amendment. Many of the current correctional health care practices originated from the 1975 Prescriptive Package, which incorporated Eighth Amendment considerations. In 1976, the U.S. Supreme Court Estelle decision further clarified that correctional facilities cannot deliberately show indifference to serious medical needs, upholding Eighth and Fourteenth Amendments of the U.S. Constitution (*Estelle v. Gamble*, 429 U.S. 97, 1976). This decision initiated rights of prisoners to health care and began to set minimal standards of health care for prisoners.

Standards for Health Services in Prison (1997) was published by the National Commission on Correctional Health Care, the national accrediting agency for correctional institutions However, specific recommendations for HIV management are not included. Specific laws related to HIV/AIDS have evolved during the past decade. Circuit courts applying Eighth Amendment rights to HIV have been divided in their rulings, leaving HIV management to the discretion of health care providers in the various correctional facilities.[37] In most cases, rulings based on "deliberate indifference"' have failed to set HIV standards of care.

The cost of providing HIV care with appropriate ART is 2–3 times more than general medical costs per offender. Initially costs of medications were reflected in limited pharmacy formularies that often excluded protease inhibitors. Over time the cost of treating with ART outweighs the costs of opportunistic diseases and declining health in HIV-infected persons not receiving ART or appropriate ART regimens.[7,11–13] Courts have failed to render unanimous opinions about which ART protocols (including protease inhibitors) correctional facilities are required to make available to HIV-infected offenders. This lack of consistency has left the issue of community standards vague. With changing professional views about the initiation and combination of ART regimens, courts make decisions that health care professionals may not support as community standards.

14. How often do prisoners become HIV-positive during incarceration?

Both sex and substance abuse occur behind bars, even though both are prohibited. According to conservative estimates, 3.2 % of offenders become HIV-infected as a result of sex and injection drug use (IDU) during incarceration.[24,38] One ex-offender in New York City told the author that he and 50 other offenders (known to be HIV-negative on entering prison) became HIV-infected while sharing one needle as part of an inmate "shooting" circle during incarceration in a state prison. HIV transmission can occur during any exchange of blood products, such as altercations involving broken skin or stabbing and tattooing with shared needles.

Sexual assault is often termed "consensual sex with intimidation" or viewed as "trading favors." Offenders may be "traded" to other prisoners or to correctional staff for sex.[25] Consent is impossible behind bars, where offenders have lost their rights and an imbalance of power exists. Offenders, especially women who lack family and social support, find themselves in a position of "swapping favors" as their only means for attaining money or goods.

15. What laws relate to sexual abuse behind bars?

The Fourth Amendment of the U.S. Constitution provides protection against sexual abuse during incarceration. This amendment states that people have the right to be secure and to be protected against unreasonable searches and seizures. Although sexual misconduct between offender and correctional officers is expressly prohibited within the federal system, this law does not bind states. Many states have enacted laws that prohibit sexual abuse and misconduct during incarceration; however, 23 states still have no such laws.[25,39]

16. Are condoms and bleach to clean syringes available in prisons?

Condoms are considered contraband, and bleach is not available to clean syringes. In the U.S. only seven correctional facilities distribute condoms: the New York City, Los Angeles County, Philadelphia, San Francisco, and Washington jails and the Vermont and Mississippi prisons.[33] These are primarily male facilities, and often the offender must proclaim himself to be homosexual to receive condoms. This practice does not help incarcerated women or men who have sex with men but do not self-identify as gay. It also has raised questions related to civil liberties. Condoms have been widely available in correctional institutions outside the U.S. As of 1997, 81% of European prison systems and the prison system of Canada have distributed condoms and reported no problems related to safety or security.[33]

Clean needles and bleach policies for IDU lag even further behind condom distribution and reflect both prison positions and philosophical debates in the U.S. about needle exchange policies.[9] Opponents argue that providing clean needles sends the message that IDU is condoned and that it is inappropriate to provide clean needles. The medical perspective acknowledges that IDU is a mental illness that contributes to transmission of sexually transmitted diseases (especially hepatitis and HIV); therefore, providing clean needles is providing good medical care.

HIV transmission behind bars can be decreased by condom and bleach distribution. Education can also reduce HIV transmission and should include universal precautions, safer sex, and proper needle cleaning. Postexposure prophylaxis (PEP) should be in place for altercations between prisoners and needlesticks that pose a possible threat of HIV infection.

17. Discuss specific issues related to the release of HIV-positive offenders.

Maintaining continuity of care and adequate medication supplies are imperative for HIV-infected offender after release. These goals are difficult to accomplish when courts release offenders early and without notice. In such circumstances, offenders leave courts without medical appointments, medications, Medicaid application, or housing. Under the best circumstances prerelease planning has created a process for meeting such needs. Correctional facilities vary in the quality of prerelease planning.

Most released offenders have difficulty maneuvering the health care system. They must have specific appointments and addresses and also must know what health care institutions have drop-in policies. Acknowledging that release brings numerous changes and adjustments and having a plan prior to release decrease missed appointments and medication doses due to lost medications and medical papers.

The ability for released offenders to engage in HIV/AIDS self-care also depends on housing and employment. Housing, employment, and prearranged medical care are imperative to ensure a successful community transition, reduce incarceration recidivism, and increase ART adherence. Housing is such a crucial component of release planning that several comprehensive residential programs are under evaluation to reduce recidivism and promote successful reentry into the community.

18. What specific programs are in place to aid HIV-infected prisoners after their release?
Under the Ryan White Comprehensive AIDS Resources Emergency (CARE) Act, federal funds supported 11 demonstration transition programs for HIV-infected offenders.[24] Each of these programs developed systematic networks of community organizations and halfway houses to maximize a successful transition. The two oldest programs are in Rhode Island (Project Bridge) and New York (Empowerment Through HIV Information, Community and Services [ETHICS], founded in 1967).[16] Both New York programs (ETHICS and Fortune Society in conjunction with Healthlink) are operated by ex-offenders.[18] These programs provide substance abuse treatment, mental health care, and comprehensive medical care, including HIV care, social support with constructive ties to the community, job readiness training, and court advocacy.

19. What resources are available for nurses and offenders in correctional facilities?
Pharmaceutical companies (many materials in Spanish and English)
• *Get Tested*, a video geared toward correctional populations (Glaxo Wellcome, Inc.)
• HIV Medication Guide (Glaxo Wecome, Inc.) of Canada, which can be downloaded at http://www.jag.on.ca)
• *Cell Wars* (Bristol-Myers Squibb Immunology), which is distributed free in a comic book format appropriate for low literacy levels and contains basic HIV information for incarcerated populations
• *A Sister's Story* (Bristol -Myers Squibb Immunology), which is distributed free in a comic book format appropriate for low literacy levels and contains basic HIV information geared toward incarcerated women
• *My Gramma Has HIV* (Agouron Pharmaceuticals)
• HIV Life Cycle Model and CD (Merck & Co.)
• Albany Medical College HIV educational series for correctional institutions in Spanish and English, with two special tapes about women's issues (telephone: 518-262-6864; e-mail: santosm@mail.amc.edu)
Newsletters
• *HEPPNews* ([HIV Education Prison Project), distributed by Brown University AIDS Program for Corrections and HIV Health Care Providers (www.hivcorrections.org)
• *HIV Inside* (distributed free by World Health CME to health care providers in correctional facilities and supported by GlaxcoWellcomeSmith (fax name and e-mail address to 212-481-8534)
HIV websites (also see bibliography)
• http:// www.hivinsite.ucsf.edu
• http://hopkins-aids.edu
• http://hiv.medscape.com
• www.amfar.org/td
• www.aidsmeds.com
• http://www.healthcg.com/hiv
• www/artis.org
• http://www.hivline.com
• http://www.cdcnac.org (Centers for Disease Control and Prevention National AIDS Clearinghouse)
• http://report.kff.org/aidshiv
• http://www.anacnet.org (Association of Nurses in AIDS Care [ANAC])

BIBLIOGRAPHY

1. AIDS Action: What Works in HIV Prevention for Incarcerated Populations. Washington DC, AIDS Action, 2001. Available at www.aidsaction.org.
2. Altice FL: Overview of HIV care. In Puisis M (ed): Clinical Practice in Correctional Medicine. St. Louis, Mosby, 1998, pp 141–163.
3. Beck AJ, Harrison PM: Prisoners in 2000. Washington, DC, U.S. Department of Justice, Bureau of Justice Statistics, 2001.
4. Beck AJ, Karlberg JC: Prison and Jail Inmates at Midyear 2000. Washington, DC, U.S. Department of Justice, Bureau of Justice Statistics, 2001.
5. Bing EG, Burnam A, Longshore D, et al: Psychiatric disorders and drug use among human immunodeficiency virus-infected adults in the United States. Arch Gen Psychiatry 58:721–728, 2001.
6. Boudin K, Carrero I, Clark J, et al: ACE: Peer education and counseling program meets the needs of incarcerated women with HIV/AIDS issues. J Assoc Nurses AIDS Care 10(6):90–98, 1999.
7. Bozzette SA, Joyce G, McCaffrey DF, et al: Expenditures for the care of HIV-infected patients in the era of highly active antiretroviral therapy. N Engl J Med 344(11):817-823, 2001.
8. Browne A, Miller B, Maguin E: Prevalence and severity of lifetime physical and sexual victimization among incarcerated women. Int J Law Psychiatry 22(3-4):301–322, 1999.
9. Buris S, Lurie P, Abrahamson JD, Rich JD: Physician prescribing of sterile injection equipment to prevent HIV infection: Time for action. Ann Intern Med 133(3):218–226, 2000.
10. Centers for Disease Control and Prevention: Prevention and control of tuberculosis in correctional facilities: Recommendations of the Advisory Council for Elimination of Tuberculosis. MMWR 45(RR-8):1–27, 1996.
11. Correctional HIV Consortium: Estimated costs for the treatment of an AIDS diagnosed inmate, 2000. Available at http://www.silcom.com/~chc/agency.html.
12. Correctional HIV Consortium: Estimated costs for the treatment of a HIV+ inmate, 2000. Available at http://www.silcom.com/~chc/agency.html.
13. DeGroot AS: HIV infection among incarcerated women: Epidemic behind bars. AIDS Reader 10(5):287–295, 2000.
14. Dole P: The feminine face of HIV. Numedex 4(1):52–53, 2002.
15. Fischl M, Rodriguez A, Sceppella E, et al: Impact of directly observed therapy on outcomes in HIV clinical trials. Programs and Abstracts of the Seventh Conference on Retroviruses and Opportunistic Infections, January 30–February 2, 2000 [abstract 71]
16. Flanigan TP, Kim JY, Zierler S, et al: A prison release program for HIV-positive women: Linking them to health services and community follow-up. J Correct Health Care 4:1–9, 1997.
17. Frank L: Prisons and public health: Emerging issues in HIV treatment adherence. J Assoc Nurses AIDS Care 10(6):25–31, 1999.
18. Freudenberg N, Wilets I, Greene MB, Richie BE: Linking women in jail to community services: Factors associated with rearrest and retention of drug-using women following release from jail. J Am Med Womens Assoc 53(2):89–93, 1998.
19. Fullilove MT, Fullilove RE, Smith M, et al: Violence, trauma, and post-traumatic stress disorder among women drug users. J Traumatic Stress 6(4):533–543, 1993.
20. Grinstead O, Zack B, Faigeles B: Collaborative research to prevent HIV among male prison inmates and their female partners. Health Educ Behav 26(2):225–238, 1999.
21. Hammett TM, Harmon P, Maruschak LM: 1994–1996 Update: HIV/AIDS, STDs, and TB in Correctional Facilities. Washington DC, U.S. Department of Justice (Office of Justice Programs), National Institute of Justice, 1997.
22. Hammett TM, Harmon P, Maruschak LM: 1996–1997 Update: HIV/AIDS, STDs, and TB in Correctional Facilities. Washington DC, U.S. Department of Justice, NCJ 176344, 1999.
23. Holzemer WL, Corless IB, Nokes KM, et al: Predictors of self-reported adherence in persons living with HIV disease. AIDS Patient Care STDS 13:185–197, 1999.
24. HRSA: Incarcerated people and HIV/AIDS. Washington DC, U.S. Department of Health and Human Services, 2000. Available at www.hrsa.gov/hab
25. Human Rights Watch Women's Rights Project: All Too Familiar: Sexual Abuse of Women in U.S. State Prisons. New York, Human Rights Watch, 1996. Available at http://www.hrw.org.
26. Jordon K, Schlenger WE, Fairbank JA, Caddell, JM: Prevalence pf psychiatric disorders among incarcerated women. Arch Gen Psychiatry 53:513–519, 1996.
27. Kantor E: AIDS and HIV infections in prisoners. AIDS Knowledge Base Website, 2001. Available at http://hivinsite.ucsf.edu/InSite.
28. Keaveny ME, Zauszniewski JA: Life events and psychological well-being in women sentenced to prison. Issues Mental Health Nurs 20:73–89, 1999.
29. Leenerts MH: The disconnected self: Consequences of abuse in a cohort of low-income white women living with HIV/AIDS. Health Care Women Int 20: 381–400, 1999.

30. Maddow R, Vernon A, Pozsik J: TB and the HIV-positive prisoner. HEPPNews 3(3), 2000. Available at www.hivcorrections.org.

31. May JP (ed): Building Violence: How America's Rush to Incarcerate Creates More Violence. Thousand Oaks, CA, Sage Publications, 2000.

32. Mostashari FM, Riley E, Selwyn PA, Altice FL: Acceptance and adherence with antiretroviral therapy among HIV-infected women in a correctional facility. J Acq Immune Defic Syndr Human Retrovirol 18: 41–348, 1998.

33. Nerenberg R: Condoms in correctional settings. HEPPNews 5(1), 2002. Available at www.hivcorrections.org.

34. Nicodemus M, Paris J: Bridging the communicable disease gap: Identifying, treating and counseling high-risk inmates. HEPPNews 4:8–9, 2001. Available at www.hivcorrections.org.

35. Roberts KJ: Physician-patient relationships, patient satisfaction, and antiretroviral medication adherence among HIV-infected adults attending a public health clinic. AIDS Patient Care STDs 16(1):43–50, 2002.

36. Rothenberg, KH, Paskey SJ: The risk of domestic violence and women with HIV infection: Implications for partner notification, public policy, and the law. Am J Public Health 85(11):1569–1575, 1995.

37. Sylla M, Thomas D: The rules, law, and AIDS in corrections. HEPPNews 3(11), 2000. Available at www.hivcorrections.org.

38. Taylor A, et al: Outbreak of HIV infection in a Scottish prison. Br J Med 310:289–292, 1995.

39. United States of America Rights for All: "Not Part of My Sentence": Violations of the Human Rights of Women in Custody. New York, Amnesty International's Campaign on the United States, 1999.

40. Vicini,J: Supreme Court upholds segregation of HIV-infected inmates. Reuters Medical News on Medscape, January 18, 2000.

41. Women's prison starts HIV education, testing. Reuters Website, 2001. Available at http://www. reutershealth.com.

24. SEVERE MENTAL ILLNESS

Jeanne K. Kemppainen, PhD, RN

Little was known about HIV/AIDS in people with severe mental illness until the early 1990s when a series of prevalence studies reported alarming rates of HIV infection, especially in people dually diagnosed with mental illness and substance abuse disorders. AIDS is now an enormous problem in mental health treatment settings and the leading cause of death among young people experiencing an initial psychiatric hospitalization.[2] Mentally ill people with HIV face the double stigma of severe mental disorder and HIV infection. Many are reluctant to seek treatment, and cases of HIV/AIDS often go unrecognized by health care providers or the persons themselves.

1. What is meant by the term *severe mental illness*?
Severe mental illness typically refers to persons with serious, persistent, and intermittent psychotic disorders, including schizophrenia, bipolar disorder, major depression, and schizoaffective disorder. These disorders have common disabling symptoms and are characterized by functional disabilities in daily living skills, social interactions, family relations, and jobs or education.[5]

2. What is the rate of HIV infection in people with severe mental illness?
Studies confirm that severely and persistently mentally ill people are at high risk for contracting HIV infection. Research shows that 1 in 12 adults diagnosed with severe mental illness is HIV-infected.[2] Seroprevalence rates vary widely across psychiatric treatment settings from 4% to 23%, with the highest infection rates in treatment programs for comorbid psychiatric and substance use disorders. Age and ethnicity distributions do not differ from nonpsychiatric groups. Women who are diagnosed with a severe mental health disorder, however, are equally as likely to be infected as men.[2]

3. How does the HIV infection rate in people with severe mental illness compare with HIV infection rates in the general population?
The overall seroprevalence rate of 8% in people with severe mental illness presents a sharp contrast in comparison with an estimated rate of 0.4% for the general population.[2] The rate of HIV/AIDS in mentally ill people is nearly 20 times higher than in persons without a psychiatric diagnosis.

4. What factors place persons with severe mental illness at increased risk for HIV/AIDS?
Severe mental disorders produce disabling cognitive, emotional, and behavioral symptoms that greatly increase the potential for HIV infection. For example, schizophrenia has a devastating impact on cognitive functioning that results in limited insight. Persons with schizophrenia frequently lack insight into their psychiatric symptoms and comprehension of their own risk for HIV/AIDS. This lack of insight also makes them much less likely to use precautions with sex or needles.[5] Mania phases of bipolar disease, on the other hand, are characterized by impulsivity, lack of judgement, reckless behavior, and increased sexual activity. Hopelessness associated with major depression results in a lack of self-care, noncompliance with treatment, and a high risk for substance use. Because apathy is a characteristic that accompanies severe mental illness, persons frequently lack the motivation to make necessary behavioral changes that reduce HIV risk.

Other important HIV risk factors relate to poverty. Many persons with severe mental illness are unable to work on a regular basis because of frequent exacerbations of their illness. As a result, they often live in dilapidated housing or homeless shelters in urban neighborhoods endemic for HIV. Sexually active people with severe mental illness who live in these areas are much more likely to be exposed to HIV-infected partners. Even when people with severe mental illness are known to have a physical disorder, many have limited access to good medical care. Problems in social functioning that contribute to HIV risk include an inability to communicate effectively or establish stable relationships with others and institutionalization in hospitals or prisons where HIV is prevalent. Between 9% and 36% of people with severe mental illness are diagnosed with one or more sexually transmitted diseases (STDs), an additional factor that increases the risk for HIV disease.

5. What about risky sexual behaviors?

Risky sexual behaviors are common among persons diagnosed with severe mental illness. The combination of disabling psychiatric symptoms and coexisting drug and alcohol disorders severely affects the ability of persons with mental illness to discriminate between safer sex practices and those that create increased risk for HIV. Risky sexual behaviors include sex with unknown partners (who are often at high risk for HIV), other psychiatric patients, multiple partners, persons with active or past injection drug use, and/or commercial sex workers. Because many persons with chronic mental illness are socioeconomically disadvantaged, they are highly susceptible to trading sex for drugs, money, a place to sleep, or basic necessities. In addition, many mentally ill men and women are forced into sex or are sexually abused. Approximately 20–40% report having sex with multiple partners, 7–28% engage in the sex trade, and 4–10% report having sex with an intravenous (IV) drug user.[1]

Communication skills needed to negotiate safe sex practices are frequently lacking, and concern about HIV risk reduction is often a low priority. Research indicates that only one-fourth of sexual encounters are protected by condom use.[1]

6. What is the association among HIV, severe mental illness, and substance abuse?

Coexisting substance use disorders are common among all major mental illnesses, including schizophrenia, major depression, bipolar disorder, and severe personality disorder. Persons with a major psychiatric diagnosis have 3 times the risk of a coexisting drug or alcohol diagnosis compared with the rest of the population. Nearly one-half of the patients diagnosed with schizophrenia meet the diagnostic criteria for substance abuse disorder.[9] Research also indicates that as many as one-third of people with a psychiatric disorder have a history of IV drug use. Since psychiatric patients who inject drugs tend to do so on an intermittent basis, this information is frequently overlooked in drug histories. The likelihood of becoming HIV-positive is increased 4-fold by crack use or sniffing drugs. A direct link also exists between substance use and unprotected sex among the severely mentally ill.[2]

7. Is there an association between the type of psychiatric diagnosis and HIV/AIDS?

Preliminary evidence suggests that people with schizophrenia or bipolar disorder are at highest risk for HIV/AIDS. The likelihood of having an HIV risk factor is also much greater if a patient has both a major psychiatric diagnosis (axis I) and a coexisting personality disorder (axis II).[8] For example, people with a major mental illness, such as bipolar disorder, and a coexisting borderline personality disorder are much less likely to use safe sex precautions during characteristic periods of emotional crises. They are also more likely to be coerced into unwanted sex. Illness severity and certain psychiatric symptoms also appear to be associated with increased HIV risk. For example, excitement symptoms related to mania are associated with "survival sex" and other high-risk sexual behaviors.[8]

8. How knowledgeable are psychiatric patients about HIV/AIDS?

In most cases, knowledge of HIV/AIDS among psychiatric patients appears to be relatively good. In studies of psychiatric patients, correct responses to AIDS knowledge questionnaires ranged from 70% to 80%.[2] This rate is comparable to that of the general population. Many persons with the most severe and disabling psychiatric disorders such as schizophrenia, however, lack key information about HIV transmission or prevention. They may possess superficial knowledge about HIV transmission but, in fact, have a limited ability to comprehend the process of HIV transmission. Because of severe cognitive deficits, they also may have difficulty in conceptualizing or understanding the implications of HIV disease and the need for treatment.

9. Discuss the important treatment considerations for people with severe mental illness and HIV/AIDS.

Providing HIV/AIDS treatment to people with severe mental illness poses many challenges and dilemmas. Besides being difficult to engage in treatment, people with severe mental illness are extremely prone to nonadherence with treatment plans or medication regimens. Cognitive deficits that accompany severe mental illness limit the ability to understand treatment recommendations and/or rationally consider the risks and benefits. Many people with severe mental illness have difficulty in explaining their symptoms to health care providers. Persons with severe psychiatric disorders may have elevated pain thresholds and, therefore, may not complain of HIV-related symptoms until the disease has progressed to a critical stage. Physical diseases are known to be more serious in patients with psychotic disorders such as schizophrenia; thus, it seems reasonable to assume that this principle may also apply to HIV-related illnesses.[10] Little information is available about the impact of severe mental illness on the clinical course of HIV/AIDS, yet anecdotal evidence suggests that patients with severe mental illness typically have poorer treatment outcomes.[10]

An important consideration in providing treatment to people with a psychiatric disorder is the integration of psychiatric and antiretroviral therapies. Although antipsychotic medications can be effectively used to treat psychiatric symptoms, even in the presence of HIV-related neurocognitive changes, these medications have the potential for adverse effects and drug-drug interactions with antiretroviral medications.[4] Generally, the lowest dose is prescribed for the shortest time possible. Patients should be observed closely for any adverse reactions. Medications used to treat depression, mania, or anxiety have fewer adverse effects.

10. What factors differentiate pre-existing mental illness from newer-onset psychiatric symptoms in people with HIV/AIDS?

Because the HIV virus is neurotropic, it crosses the blood-brain barrier and enters the central nervous system (CNS) shortly after infection. CNS manifestations resulting from HIV infection include HIV-related dementia, psychotic disorders, CNS opportunistic infections and tumors, encephalophathies linked to systemic or metabolic conditions, mood disorders, and delirium. Persons without a previous history of mental illness may develop psychiatric symptoms as a result of these HIV-related disorders.[7] Distinguishing between HIV-related disorders and pre-existing mental illness is often difficult and involves a complete medical evaluation and neuopsychological testing. An important nursing contribution includes a thorough assessment of functional and psychosocial status. Pharmacologic interventions for people with newer-onset psychiatric symptoms are similar to those used in people with pre-existing mental illness.[7] However, treatment is aimed primarily at correcting the underlying medical complications.

11. How does severe mental illness influence adherence to antiretroviral therapies?

Adherence to prescribed medications and treatments is a continuing problem for people with severe mental illness. The mean level of adherence is 58% for psychotropic medicines and 63% for antidepressants.[3] The most frequently cited reasons for nonadherence to psychiatric medicines are as follows:

• Difficulty in accepting a diagnosis of mental illness and the need for treatment
• Stigma of mental illness
• History of substance use
• Unpleasant medication side-effects

The added requirements of the rigorous and complex regimens that frequently accompany antiretroviral therapies create a challenging dimension to the care and treatment of patients with severe mental illness. Because they have such great difficulty in adhering to medication regimens, there is widespread concern about the ability of patients with severe mental illness to maintain antiretroviral therapy. Recent findings show that persons with schizophrenia use antiretroviral drugs more consistently than other patients. This may reflect greater involvement with health care providers related to their chronic illnesses.[10]

12. What actions should the nurse take in relation to medication adherence?

Helping the client with severe mental illness to understand medication significance is an important nursing intervention. Because many people with severe and persistent mental illness may not understand that they are ill and require medication, its important to evaluate their attitudes, beliefs, and past experiences with both psychiatric and HIV medication regimens. People with mental illness may place a greater priority on one medication regimen or the other or may regard all medication as unpleasant or unnecessary. They may also be taking medications in a way different from the way in which they were prescribed. The nurse should evaluate the person's ability to understand dosages and medication schedules and ability to self-administer medicines or fill prescriptions. Medication teaching programs should be tailored to reflect the cognitive limitations presented by patients with severe mental illness.

13. What types of HIV/AIDS education programs are most effective for the mentally ill?

People with severe mental illness, especially those who live on the streets, are unlikely to take advantage of traditional HIV/AIDS prevention programs. Prevention programs that rely primarily on brief, "quick-fix" interventions for distributing information, such as the use of pamphlets or lectures, have been found to have little influence on modifying the HIV/AIDS risk behaviors of psychiatric patients. Street-based outreach and culturally tailored, intensive, small-group programs that simultaneously target knowledge, attitudes, motivation, and cognitive and behavioral skills are much more effective at reducing HIV risk, even among people with long histories of severe mental illness.[6]

14. Which HIV prevention strategies are most effective for people with chronic mental illness?

Health providers have found that people with severe mental illness can tolerate and benefit from frank discussions of HIV risk behaviors. Interpersonal and social skills related to HIV risk reduction can also be improved through individual and group teaching.[6] People with severe mental illness respond positively when a variety of teaching strategies aimed at overcoming cognitive deficits are used. For example, the combination of pictures and oral problem-solving is highly effective in discussing high-risk situations. Because many people with severe mental illness base HIV risk potential only on the outward physical appearance of other people, interventions should be tailored to help them focus on their own risk behaviors. Intensive skills training also needs to be a central component of HIV risk reduction training.[6]

15. What approach should a nurse take if she or he suspects that a client with severe mental illness has HIV disease?

A nurse who notes physical signs suggestive of HIV/AIDS should report his or her observations to the appropriate providers. A thorough assessment of the person's knowledge about HIV infection and any high-risk behaviors helps to form an essential basis for clinical decision-making about HIV testing. Providers should always refer patients for HIV testing when a potential diagnosis of HIV/AIDS is suspected or when a patient presents symptoms suggestive of CNS dysfunction. Before a decision is made to test a person with mental illness, however, his or her capacity for providing informed consent must be determined. Voluntary testing is encouraged. People with mental illness should be able to complete counseling and HIV testing without an increase in psychiatric symptoms. They may, however, require more than a single pre- or post-test counseling session.

BIBLIOGRAPHY

1. Carey M, Carey K, Kalichman S: Risk for human immunodeficiency virus (HIV) infection among persons with severe mental illness. Clin Psychol Rev 17(3):271–291, 1997.
2. Cournos F, McKinnon K, Rosner J: HIV among individuals with severe mental illness. Psychiatr Ann 31(1):50–56, 2001.
3. Cramer JA, Rosencheck R: Compliance with medication regimens for mental and physical disorders. Psychiatr Serv 49(2):196–201, 1998.
4. Ferrando SJ, Khakasa W: Psychopharmacological treatment of patients with HIV and AIDS. Psychiatr Q 73(1):33–49, 2002.
5. Johnson DL: Overview of severe mental illness. Clin Psychol Rev 17(3):247–257, 1997.
6. Kelly J: HIV risk reduction intervention for persons with severe mental illness. Clin Psychol Rev 17(3):293–309, 1997.
7. McDonald JS, Purcell DW, Farber EW: Severe mental illness and HIV-related medical and neuropsychiatric sequelae. Clin Psychol Rev 17(3):311–325, 1997.
8. Otto-Salaj LL, Stevenson LY: Influence of psychiatric diagnosis and symptoms on HIV risk behavior in adults with serious mental illness. AIDS Reader 11(4):197–208, 2001.
9. Regier DA, Boyd JH, Burke JD, et al: One-month prevalence of mental disorders in the United States: Based on five epidemiologic catchment area sites. Arch Gen Psychiatry 45:977–986, 1988.
10. Walkup J, Sambamoorthi U, Crystal S: Incidence and consistency and antiretroviral use among HIV-infected Medicaid beneficiaries with schizophrenia. J Clin Psychiatry 62(3):174–178, 2001.

GLOSSARY

Access to care: availability of services, including time, cost, distance, and appropriateness.

Acquired immunodeficiency syndrome (AIDS): CD4 count equal to or less than 200 counts/mm^3 in the presence of HIV and/or the presence of an AIDS-defining illness.

Adherence: all activities necessary to achieve the most positive outcome for each patient.

Aggregate HIV housing: placing HIV inmates in a separate facility from other inmates.

AIDS: *See* Acquired immunodeficiency syndrome.

Allele: paired gene with specific inheritable traits that positions itself on a paired chromosome.

Anabolic steroid: testosterone or steroid hormone that stimulates anabolism.

Anabolism: metabolic phase involving the building of body substances and the repair and growth of cells.

Anergy: lost or weakened body response to an antigen administered by skin test; opposite of allergy, an overreaction to an allergen.

Anthropometric: referring to measurement of the human body and its parts.

Antiretroviral therapy (ART): use of drugs to combat retroviruses (e.g., HIV).

ART: *See* Antiretroviral therapy.

Arthralgia: joint pain.

Assay: analysis of a substance to determine its components and their proportion of the whole.

Aspergillus: a species of fungus. *Aspergillus fumigatus*, found in soil and water, is the most frequent cause of infection in humans and birds.

Autonomy: ethical principle that focuses on the right of competent people to make informed decisions related to their lives and treatments.

Ayurveda: an ancient/modern Indian system of achieving and maintaining health and spiritual growth. Treatments include purgatives, periodic fasting, proper diet, herbs and food, meditation, aromatherapy, self-massage, and regular daily routines.

Body habitus changes: altered physical appearance (e.g., peripheral fat wasting, fat redistribution).

Beneficence: ethical principle that means "do good;" corollary of nonmaleficence.

Bipolar disorder: illness characterized by manic and/or manic and depressive phases.

Cachexia: generalized ill health, wasting, and malnutrition, frequently related to serious disease.

CAM: *See* Complementary alternative medicine/therapy.

Candidiasis: fungal, yeast infection of skin and mucous membranes, especially the mouth, esophagus, bronchi, lungs, and/or vagina.

CAT: *See* Complementary alternative medicine/therapy.

Catabolism: metabolic phase involving the breakdown of complex substances in the body into simpler components. Energy is frequently released in the process.

CD4 (T4 or T helper cells): T cell involved in immune response that signals other cells to respond to viral, protozoan, and fungal infections. HIV attaches to CD4 receptor molecules, interferes with the immune response, and results in decreased CD4 counts.

Coccidioidomycosis: fugal infection beginning in the respiratory tract that can spread throughout the body (disseminated).

Chorioretinitis: choroid and retinal inflammation, frequently caused by cytomegalovirus. It may be asymptomatic, have early unilateral floaters and decreased visual acuity, and progress to bilateral disease and blindness.

CMV: *See* Cytomegalovirus.

Coasting period: temporary increase in distal peripheral neuropathy (DPN) symptoms after stopping drugs that cause DPN.

Comorbidity: the existence of a secondary disease in the presence of a primary disease.

Complementary and alternative medicine (CAM)/therapy (CAT): combination of the terms that refers to health treatments, approaches, and philosophies that are outside the paradigm of traditional Western medicine/therapeutics.

Compliance: following instructions given by someone "who knows better" (paternalistic connotation).

Confidentiality: ethical principle and legal responsibility whereby the health care provider must respect the client's privacy and share with persons who have a right to know only the information about the client that they need to know.

Consensual sex with intimidation: sexual assault or trading sexual favors behind bars, where consent is impossible because of loss of rights and imbalance of power.

Cryptococcal meningitis: infection of the meninges of the brain and spinal column with cryptococci.

Cryptococcosis: fungal infection, usually in the respiratory tract or brain, that may affect any body part; transmitted through soil containing contaminated bird droppings.

Cryptosporidiosis: protozoan infection of the gastrointestinal tract, causing diarrhea; transmitted by contaminated food and water.

Cultural competence: the ability to perform professional tasks effectively for all different racial, ethnic, linguistic, and cultural groups that access services.

Cytokine: protein produced by white blood cells to mediate (increase or decrease) inflammatory and immune responses.

Cytomegalovirus (CMV): herpes virus that causes chorioretinitis and pneumonia in immuno-compromised people.

Deontology: ethical theory that focuses on duty and the consistent application of principles in all situations. People are ends versus means to an end.

Directly observed therapy (DOT): policy that requires patients to take medications under direct supervision. In prisons the frequency of doses can reveal the HIV status of the inmate and lead to stigmatization.

Disclosure: an encompassing term that refers to revealing or exposing information about a person; includes self-disclosure.

Discordant couple: a couple consisting of one HIV-infected partner and one uninfected partner.

Discrimination: unfair or unequal treatment or withholding of privileges because of demographic variables.

Disseminated: distributed throughout an organ or the body.

Distal peripheral neuropathy (DPN): damage to peripheral nerves; possible side effect of certain medications.

Dope houses: buildings where drugs are sold and injected. *See* Shooting galleries.

DOT: *See* Directly observed therapy.

DPN: *See* Distal peripheral neuropathy.

Duty to care: ethical principle that requires health care providers to provide treatment regardless of the person's demographic variables and diagnosis.

Dysesthesia: abnormal skin sensations, such as numbness, tingling, prickling, and burning; paresthesia.

Dyslipidemia: metabolic complication with abnormal cholesterol and triglyceride blood values.

Dysmorphic: deformed.

EIA: *See* Enzyme immune assay.

ELISA: *See* Enzyme-linked immunosorbent assay.

End-of-life issues: factors related to planning for death, including decisions about caretakers, living will, health care proxy, power of attorney, will, and care for dependents.

Enteropathy: disease of the intestinal tract.

Enzyme Immunoassay (EIA): screening test for hepatitis C virus (HCV). EIA detects antibodies to HCV but does not differentiate among acute, chronic, or resolved infection.

Enzyme-linked immunosorbent assay (ELISA): enzyme immunoassay of blood and/or body fluids for the presence of HIV antibodies; a screening test.

Epidemic: disease present in a large number of people in a geographic area.

Ergot derivative: drug developed from fungus that can cause vasoconstriction and spasm; should not be used with protease inhibitors.

Ethics: morality or good of human conduct.

Female circumcision: removal of part or all of the clitoris, usually before puberty; practiced in females from some African and Mid-Eastern and Far-Eastern cultures.

Female genital mutilation (FGM): removal of the clitoris, prepuce, labia minora, and sometimes labia majora, usually before puberty; practiced in females from some African, Mid-Eastern, and Southeastern Asian cultures.

FGM: *See* Female genital mutilation.

Fixing dates: transactions of sex for drugs or transactions when the sex worker "shoots up" (injects) with the client.

Genome: complete genetic information of a cell; all genes in the chromosomes.

Genotype: genetic/hereditary composition of an organism.

Genotypic (resistance) assay: test to determine a person's resistance to current antiretroviral drug.

HAART: *See* Highly active antiretroviral therapy.

HAD: *See* HIV-associated dementia and metabolic encephalopathy.

Harm reduction model: value-neutral approach that accepts the reality that drug use continues and includes initiatives to minimize danger to all (e.g., needle exchange, condoms).

HCV RNA PCR: *See* Hepatitis C virus RNA polymerase chain reaction.

Hepatitis C virus RNA polymerase chain reaction (HCV RNA PCR): assay used to detect HCV in severely immunocompromised persons (CD4 > 100 cells/mm^3).

Highly active antiretroviral therapy (HAART): combination of three or more drugs for aggressive reduction of viral load and HIV progression.

Histoplasmosis: fungal infection, acquired by inhaling spores, that progresses from the respiratory tract throughout the body.

HIV: *See* Human immunodeficiency virus.

HIV-associated dementia (HAD): *See* Metabolic encephalopathy.

Homeopathic medicine: use of small amounts of drug to cure a disease caused by large amounts of the same drug.

HPV: *See* Human papilloma virus.

Human immunodeficiency virus (HIV): retrovirus infection, spread primarily through blood and sexual contact; causes acquired immunodeficiency syndrome (AIDS).

Human papilloma virus (HPV): viral infection, spread through sexual contact, that causes genital warts and is associated with cervical and other genital cancers.

Humoral immunity: immunity based on antibody production in body fluids (e.g., plasma, lymph).

IDU: *See* Injection drug user.

Immunocompetent: having an intact immune system.

Immunocompromised: having an impaired immune system with decreased ability to resist infections and tumors. *See* Immunodeficient.

Immunodeficient: having an impaired immune system with decreased ability to resist infections and tumors. *See* Immunocompromised.

Immunosuppressed: blocked from activating an immune response.

Incidence: the number of people acquiring a disease in a population in a given period of time (e.g., the number of people newly infected with HIV in New York City during 2001).

Infectivity: probability of transfer of an organism from an infected to an uninfected person after an exposure; organism's ability to enter host and replicate.[3]

Informed consent: the client's voluntary agreement to a plan based on clear, understandable information.

Informed refusal: the client's voluntary nonacceptance of a plan based on clear, understandable information.

Injection drug user (IDU): inclusive term for all people who inject substances, intravenously (IV), intramuscularly (IM), and/or subcutaneously (SC). This term is synonymous with the term *injecting drug user* and replaces the more limiting term, *intravenous drug user* (IVDU).

Intravenous drug user (IVDU): *See* Injection drug user (IDU).

In vitro: testing in the laboratory versus testing in the living organism (in vivo).

Isosporiasis: protozoan infection of the gastrointestinal tract, causing diarrhea; thought to be transmitted by direct contact with contaminated water or infected people or animals.

IVDU: *See* Intravenous and injection drug user.

Justice: the ethical principle of fairness in general and in the distribution of resources.

Kaposi's sarcoma (KS): cancerous lesion(s) of the skin and internal body, thought to be caused by the human herpesvirus-8. Its characteristic lesion is firm and purple to brown-black and does not blanch when pressed.

Keep on person (KOP): prison policy that allows inmates to hold medications and take them without direct supervision. This practice promotes confidentiality.

KOP: *See* Keep on person.

KS: *See* Kaposi's sarcoma.

Lactacidemia/lacticemia/lactic acidosis: spectrum of excessive lactic acid in the blood.

Legal: based in statutes, laws, or legislation.

LIGHT model of care: personalized nursing interventions to assist client in independent decision-making and actions.

Lipoatrophy: fat wasting.

Lipodystrophy: fat metabolism disturbance, including fat wasting, accumulation, and/or redistribution.

Lipodystrophy syndrome: group of metabolic and morphologic symptoms and complications that may or may not be part of a single clinical syndrome.

Lipohypertrophy: fat accumulation or redistribution.

Lochia: blood, tissue, and mucus discharged after birth.

Lymphokines: nonantibody proteins (cytokines), such as gamma interferon and interleukins, produced by lymphatic cells to stimulate an immune response.

Lymphoma: neoplasm of lymphoid tissue, usually malignant. Names of tumors relate to the site involved (e.g., central nervous system) or person who described them first (e.g., Hodgkin's).

MAC/MAI: *See Mycobacterium avium* and *Mycobacterium intracellulare.*

Maleficence: the act of doing harm; opposite of beneficence.

MDR TB: *See* Multiple drug/multidrug-resistant tuberculosis.

Meningitis: inflammation of the membranes of the brain and spinal column. The most common organisms associated with persons with HIV/AIDS are *Cryptococcus neoformans*, cytomegalovirus, other herpes viruses, and *Toxoplasma gondii.*

Metabolic: referring to all physical and chemical changes in a body.

Metabolic encephalopathy: altered brain consciousness or function, resulting from failure of other organs; HIV-associated dementia (HAD).

Monotherapy: treatment with one drug.

Morphologic: referring to the structure and form of an organism, not its function.

mTB: *Mycobacterium tuberculosis.*

Mucocutaneous: referring to mucous membranes and skin; route of HIV exposure (e.g., infant during vaginal birth).

Multiple drug/multidrug resistant tuberculosis (MDR-TB): TB organism that does not respond to two or more of the usual TB-specific pharmacologic agents.

Myalgia: muscle pain or soreness.

***Mycobacterium avium* (MAC) and *Mycobacterium intracellulare* (MAI):** atypical mycobacteria, found in soil and water, that cause pulmonary and systemic disease in immunocompromised people.

***Mycobacterium tuberculosis* (mTB):** one of the earliest opportunistic infections, transmitted by aerosolized droplets. The organism lodges primarily in the respiratory tract but may affect other body areas.

Myopathy: disorder of striated muscle, usually characterized by progressive weakness.

Naive: referring both to a *person* who has had no experience with HIV drugs and to *T cells* designed to react to specific antigens.

Needle exchange program (NEP): at the minimum, replacing used needles with new ones. Additional services and supports for IDUs may include:HIV and hepatitis testing, immunization, counseling, and reinforcement of prevention measures.

NEP: *See* Needle exchange program.

Neuropathy: disorder of the nerves ranging from paresthesia to paralysis.

NHL: *See* Non-Hodgkin's lymphoma.

NNRTI: *See* Nonnucleoside reverse transcriptase inhibitor.

Non-Hodgkin's lymphoma (NHL): most prevalent lymphoma associated with HIV/AIDS, usually involving the central nervous system, gastrointestinal tract, liver, and bone marrow.

Nonmaleficence: ethical principle that means "do not harm;" a corollary of beneficence.

Nonnucleoside reverse transcriptase inhibitor (NNRTI): drug that binds with the HIV-1 reverse transcriptase site; has additive effect with other drugs.

NRTI: *See* Nucleoside reverse transcriptase inhibitor.

Nucleoside reverse transcriptase inhibitor (NRTI): antiretroviral drug that suppresses replication of the retrovirus by prematurely terminating its proviral chain.

Odynophagia: painful swallowing.

OI: *See* Opportunistic infection.

Oligodendrocyte: neuroglial cell, originating in the ectoderm, that connects and supports tissue and is a major factor in the nervous system's response to injury and infection.

Opportunistic infection (OI): usually a latent, sometimes a new, infection that emerges as the immune system is weakened (e.g., through chronic infection with HIV, cancer, chemotherapy).

Osteopenia: decreased amount of bone tissue.

OTC: *See* Over the counter.

Over the counter (OTC): drugs that can be purchased without a prescription (e.g., analgesics and antacids).

Palliative care: client- and family-centered approach to relieving symptoms versus curing disease, usually near the end of life. The focus is on the quality not the quantity of life.

Pancrelipase: a combination of enzymes, mostly lipases, used to treat pancreatic secretion deficiencies.

Pancytopenia: decrease of all cells in the blood.

Pandemic: widespread disease in a country or region or throughout the world.

Parentalism: term used interchangeably with paternalism to avoid gender bias; refers to the belief that the provider can decide what information should be shared with the patient and knows best about health decisions. *See* Paternalism.

Paresthesia: abnormal sensation, including numbness, tingling, prickling, burning, pins and needles.

Paternalism: belief that the provider can decide what information should be shared with the patient and knows best about health decisions. *See* Parentalism.

PCP: *See Pneumocystis carinii* pneumonia.

PCR: *See* Polymerase chain reaction.

Pegulated interferon: alpha interferon with a glycol attachment to increase its antiviral activity.

PEP: *See* Postexposure prophylaxis.

Perinatal transmission: transfer of organism across the placenta, during labor and delivery, and/or through breast milk.

Phenotype: manifestation of genes in an organism noted by direct observation or through tests.

Phenotypic (resistance) assay: DNA test of HIV to determine its sensitivity to an antiretroviral drug.

PI: *See* Protease inhibitor.

PML: *See* Progressive multifocal leukoencephalopathy.

***Pneumocystis carinii* pneumonia (PCP):** possible fungal infection, spread by inhalation of the cyst form of the organism. This most common opportunistic infection for people with HIV/AIDS usually affects the respiratory system but can involve the skin, eye, heart, liver, and spleen.

Polymerase chain reaction (PCR): laboratory procedure involving rapid replication of genetic material that can be tested for presence of certain bacteria, viruses (e.g., HIV), and diseases; measures viral load.

Postexposure prophylaxis (PEP): use of combination of antiretroviral drugs to reduce the risk of HIV infection after exposure to blood or body fluids of a person infected with HIV.

PPD: *See* Purified protein derivative.

Prevalence: the total number of people or percent of the population of an area affected by a particular disease (e.g., the total number of people infected with HIV in New York State in 2001).

Primary central nervous system (CNS) lymphoma: major malignant neoplasm in persons with HIV/AIDS.

Privacy: the right of a person to control what, where, and when his or her personal information is shared.

Probity: honesty, integrity.

Progressive multifocal leukoencephalopathy (PML): JC viral opportunistic infection of the brain and spinal cord, with rapid degeneration and death.

Protease inhibitor (PI): antiviral drug that blocks the action of the protease enzyme and prevents viral replication.

Proteolysis: breakdown of protein into simpler substances, usually involving enzyme action.

Psychotropic: affecting mental abilities, including behavior.

Purified protein derivative (PPD): contents of the intradermal (tuberculin skin) test for tuberculosis, frequently used as the name of the test.

Qi gong: Chinese martial art that uses movement, breathing, and meditation for the development of relaxation, strength, flexibility, and concentration.

Recombinant human growth hormone: altered hormone to produce increased effect.

Recombinant immunoblot assays (RIBAs): tests used to confirm a questionable diagnosis of hepatitis C.

Refractory: resistant to stimulation (nerve or muscle) or usual treatment.

Retrovirus: virus containing reverse transcriptase that produces a DNA molecule from an RNA molecule (e.g., HIV).

Reverse transcriptase inhibitor (RTI): drug that interferes with the reverse transcriptase viral stage (production of DNA molecule from RNA molecule).

RIBA: *See* Recombinant immunoblot assay.

RTI: *See* Reverse transcriptase inhibitor.

Sanctity of life: ethical principle referring to the belief in the inherent worth of each person.

Seroprevalence: proportion of persons who have positive serum tests of an infection (e.g., HIV) at a certain time.

Seroreverter: child who was born to an HIV-positive mother but shows no signs of HIV infection.

Severe mental illness: serious, persistent, and intermittent psychotic disorders, including schizophrenia, bipolar disorder, major depression, and schizoaffective disorders.

Sex trade workers: women or men who participate in sexual activity for money or drugs; replaces the term *prostitute*.

Sexually transmitted disease (STD): general term denoting any of approximately 25 infections transmitted by direct sexual contact; formerly called *venereal disease* (VD).

Shooting galleries: apartments or houses where drugs are sold and injected. *See* Dope houses.

Silencing the self: women's suppression of feelings, thoughts, and actions in order to adhere to society's expectations. The Silencing the Self Scale[4] has four subscales that measure judging self by external standards, putting needs of others before self, withholding responses to avoid conflict, and resenting an external self that does not reflect one's anger and hostility.

Social context: for injection drug users, the aggregate of social and physical factors determining the milieu for injection drug use and HIV risk in a geographic area. Components include the users, shooting gallery, drug dealers, and time of initiation.

STD: *See* Sexually transmitted disease.

Steroid psychosis: mental disorder characterized by reality disorientation and personality changes; caused by steroid therapy.

Strongyloidosis: infestation with the filiform larvae of roundworms found in the soil and transmitted through the skin to the blood, lungs, and intestinal tract.

Support framework for women: Friedman's[1] concepts related to individual and family behaviors: coherence (sustaining unity/connectedness), maintenance (promoting stability and control), change (testing values and setting new priorities), and individuation (searching for meaningful existence).

Syncytial virus: a term referring to viruses with contiguous protoplasm.

Tai chi: Chinese martial art that uses slow, controlled movements to develop relaxation, balance, strength, flexibility, and concentration.

Teleology: ethical theory that focuses on outcomes of actions in light of the greatest good for the greatest number. People may be a means to achieve a goal rather than an end in themselves. *See* Utilitarianism.

Teratogenic: causing defects in an embryo; potential side effect of certain drugs.

Toxoplasma gondii **(Toxo):** protozoan infection, transmitted through uncooked meat of infected birds or animals and cat feces, that affects the brain, lungs, liver, and other body organs.

Traditional Chinese medicine: holistic medical system that focuses on the balance of energy and opposites within the body.

Tropism: involuntary reaction of an organism toward or from an external stimulus.

Trucking: the use of trucks in transportation. In Africa the prevalence of HIV/AIDS frequently is related to truck routes, linking truck drivers, sex workers, and HIV/AIDS.

Utilitarianism: ethical theory that focuses on outcomes of actions in light of the greatest good for the greatest number. People may be a means to achieve a goal rather than an end in themselves. *See* Teleogy.

Veracity: ethical principle that refers to truth-telling and honesty in communication; opposite of paternalism/parentalism.

Viral load: amount of HIV in the blood, reported as "copies."

Viral suppression: interference with HIV replication, resulting in decreased viral loads.

Viremia: virus in the blood.

Virilization: masculine secondary sex characteristics in a woman.

Virion: genome in a protective protein coat; a matured virus.

Virologic test: test for a specific virus.

Vpr: HIV-1 gene coded for proteins involved in activating transcription.

Vpu: HIV-1 gene coded for proteins needed for viral budding.

Wasting: involuntary weight loss with depletion of lean tissue, resulting in loss of strength and muscle size; frequently associated with fever and diarrhea.

Western blot assay: sensitive antibody test used to confirm two positive ELISAs for HIV.

Yang: Chinese complementary concept of light, male, sun.

Yin: Chinese complementary concept of dark, female, moon.

Yi-yang: Chinese opposing and complementary concepts that are brought to balance in traditional Chinese medicine.

BIBLIOGRAPHY

1. Friedemann ML: The Framework of Systemic Organization: A Conceptual Approach to Families and Nursing. Thousand Oaks, CA, Sage, 1995.
2. Glossary of HIV/AIDS-Related Terms, 3rd ed. Washington, DC, HIV/AIDS Treatment Information Service, 1999.
3. Harkness GA: Epidemiology in Nursing Practice. St. Louis, Mosby, 1995.
4. Jack DC: Silencing the Self: Women and Depression. New York, Harper Collins, 1991
5. Ropka ME, Williams AB: HIV Nursing and Symptom Management. Boston, Jones & Bartlett, 1998.
6. Ungvarski PJ, Flaskerud JH: HIV/AIDS: A Guide to Primary Care Management, 4th ed. Philadelphia, W.B. Saunders, 1999.
7. Venes D (ed.): Taber's Cyclopedic Medical Dictionary, 19th ed. Philadelphia, F. A. Davis, 2001.

INDEX

Page numbers in **boldface type** indicate complete chapters.